Mammography for Radiologic Technologists

Mammography for Radiologic Technologists

Second Edition

Gini Wentz, RT,(R) (M)

Breast Imaging Specialist
West Orange, New Jersey

with

WARD C. PARSONS, MD, RT

Susan B. Koman Breast Center
St. Francis Hospital
Peoria, Illinois

McGraw-Hill   **Health Professions Division**
New York   St. Louis   San Francisco   Auckland   Bogotá   Caracas   Lisbon   London   Madrid
Mexico City   Milan   Montreal   New Delhi   Paris   San Juan   Singapore   Sydney   Tokyo   Toronto

McGraw-Hill

A Division of The McGraw·Hill Companies

Mammography for Radiologic Technologists, 2/e

1234567890 QPKQPK 9876

ISBN 0-07-105845-1

This book was set in Caledonia by York Graphic Services, Inc.
The editors were J.T. Morgan and P. McCurdy. The production supervisor was Rick Ruzycka. The indexer was Irving C. Tullar.
Quebecor/Kingsport was printer and binder.

This book is printed on acid-free paper.

Cataloging-in-publication data is on file for this book at the Library of Congress.

To Edwin C. and Betty F. Wentz, who served as Lutheran missionaries in Japan for 40 years, and to our peers, who have made the commitment to ensure that women will always obtain the best mammograms possible.

Contents

1 History of Mammography   1

2 Overview of Mammography   7

3 Anatomy and Physiology of the Breast   11

4

The Image   17

5

What Mammography Means to the Patient and the Technologist   37

8

Special Procedures in Mammography   85

9

Quality Assurance and Quality Control   93

10 Troubleshooting Guide 123

List of Abbreviations

ACR—American College of Radiology

ACS—American Cancer Society

AEC—automatic exposure control

Al—aluminum

ARRT—American Registry of Radiologic Technologists

BCDDP—Breast Cancer Detection Demonstration Project

Be—beryllium

B + F—base plus fog

BSE—breast self-examination

CC—craniocaudal

CGR—Company of General Radiography (U.S. name), Compagnie Générale de Radiologie (French name)

CIS—carcinoma in situ

cm—centimeters

DCIS—disseminated carcinoma in situ

dd—density difference

FDA—Food and Drug Administration

FNA—fine needle aspiration

H&D curve—Hurter and Driffield, characteristic curve, or sensitometric curve

HCFA—Healthcare Finance Act

HIP—Health Insurance Plan

HVL—half-value layer

in—inches

kVp—kilovoltage peak

lb—pounds

LIQ—lower inner quadrant

LM—lateromedial

LOQ—lower outer quadrant

mA—milliamperes

mAs—milliampere-seconds

md—mid-density

min—minutes

ML—mediolateral

MLO—mediolateral oblique

mm—millimeters

Mo—molybdenum

MQSA—Mammography Quality Standards Act

OR—operating room

PM—preventive maintenance

PQC—processor quality control

PT—phototimer

QA—quality assurance

QC—quality control

R—radiation

RSNA—Radiologic Society of North America

s—seconds

SID—source-to-image distance

TDLU—terminal ductal lobular unit

TLD—thermoluminescent dosimeter

UIQ—upper inner quadrant

UOQ—upper outer quadrant

UV—ultraviolet

W—tungsten

List of Figures

Foreword

Mammography is one of the great ongoing success stories of medicine in the twentieth century. Originally developed as a diagnostic method to evaluate patients referred for palpable breast masses, it is now more commonly used to screen asymptomatic women for clinically unsuspected breast cancer. Here lies its major value, since recent studies suggest that annual mammographic screening could reduce the breast cancer death rate by as much as 50%.[1,2]

Such results are possible due to dramatic improvements in dedicated mammographic units,[3,4] film-screen systems,[5] and processors that have occurred over the past 20 years, which allow for much higher quality images than previously possible. Yet attainment of optimal mammographic quality images requires not only state-of-the-art equipment but also proper application in terms of breast positioning, compression, technique selection, and quality control. New mammographic views and breast positioning methods allow better visualization than ever before but require greater technical knowledge and skills.[6,7] Increased emphasis on quality control[8] ensures consistently optimal functioning of mammographic units and film processors but presents additional challenges to the technologist.

The better the quality of the mammography at an office, clinic, or hospital, the larger the number of early cancers that will be detected and the more lives that will be saved from breast cancer among the women screened there. However, the quality of mammography may vary considerably from one facility to another.[9] That is why it is so important to attain high-quality mammography throughout our country by means of such recent endeavors as the American College of Radiology (ACR) Mammography Accreditation Program[10] and the American Registry of Radiologic Technologists (ARRT) Mammography Subspecialty Examination.[11]

Mammography for Radiologic Technologists, by Gini Wentz, RT, with Ward C. Parsons, MD, represents a significant contribution to these efforts. Ms.

[1]Feig SA. Decreased breast cancer mortality through mammographic screening, results of clinical trials. Radiology 1988;167:659–665.

[2]Feig SA, Ehrlich SM. Estimation of radiation risk from screening mammography: recent trends and comparison with expected benefits. Radiology 1990;174:638–647.

[3]Feig SA. Mammography equipment: Principles, features, selection. Radiol Clin North Am 1987;25:897–911.

[4]Conway BJ, McCrohan JL, Rueter FG, Suleiman OH, Mammography in the eighties. Radiology 1990;177:335–339.

[5]Feig SA. Screen-film mammography systems, processing and dedicated units. Syllabus for the Categorical Course on Breast Imaging, September 22–23, 1990. Reston, VA: American College of Radiology; 1990:1–10.

[6]Sickles EA. Practical solutions to common mammographic problems: Tailoring the examination. AJR 1988;151:31–39.

[7]Feig SA. Importance of supplementary views to diagnostic accuracy. AJR 1988;151:40–41.

[8]American College of Radiology Committee on Quality Assurance in Mammography. Mammography Quality Control, Radiologic Technologists Manual. Reston, VA: American College of Radiology; 1990.

[9]Galkin BM, Feig SA, Muir HD. The technical quality of mammography in centers participating in a regional breast cancer awareness program. Radiographics 1988;8:133–145.

[10]Hendrick RE. Standardization of image quality and radiation dose in mammography. Radiology 1990;174:648–654.

[11]ARRT presents new exam project updates. ARRT Newsletter. Mendota Heights, MN: ARRT; August 1990.

Wentz is uniquely qualified to have written this text. A former Coordinator of Applications and Medical Education in Mammography for Thompson–CGR Medical Corporation, Territory Sales Manager for Fuji Medical Systems USA, and currently Technical Applications and Product Manager in Mammography for AGFA Corporation, she has extensive experience in the development, production, marketing, and sale of mammographic equipment and film. She has trained numerous mammography technologists across the United States during on-site customer-training sessions, technical workshops, and lectures. As the need for one-on-one training became greater than Gini could handle by herself during her 7-day-a-week, cross-country itinerary, she designed and conducted mammography training programs for her company's technical specialists so that they, in turn, could teach their customers. On the national level, she rapidly became known to leading radiologists and technologists as a valued consultant and "troubleshooter" in the technical aspects of mammography. By virtue of these activities she has made a substantial contribution to bettering the quality of mammographic studies across the country.

The route by which Gini Wentz became involved in mammography is interesting. Born into a family whose roots were in rural southeastern Pennsylvania, she grew up in Japan, where her parents have worked for over 40 years as Lutheran missionaries. After Gini completed her early schooling there (she is fluent in Japanese), she returned to the United States for further education at York College in York, Pennsylvania, and Roanoke College in Salem, Virginia, later graduating from the School of Radiologic Technology at Carlisle Hospital in Carlisle, Pennsylvania. During her 11 years of work experience as a staff technologist and assistant administrative technologist at Gettysburg Hospital in Gettysburg, Pennsylvania, she developed an interest in mammography that led to a new job as a mammography product specialist with Thompson-CGR Corporation. There she quickly became a key member of their corporate team, which captured 40% of the United States mammography market sales. Although her extraordinary career in mammography was not a predictable course for the daughter of Lutheran missionaries to the Far East, she has in a sense been a missionary herself in bringing the lifesaving benefits of mammography to hundreds of thousands of women in her own country.

This textbook represents a further extension of Gini Wentz's teaching activities for mammographic technologists, allowing her to reach an even wider audience. It contains much practical information culled from the author's many years of interactions with manufacturers, representatives, technologists, medical physicists, chemists, engineers, radiologists, and, last but not least, patients. It should further educate technologists, enabling them to produce high-quality mammograms that they can take pride in. Mammography, in and of itself, does not produce uniformly excellent results, regardless of how the procedure is performed. Rather, it is an imaging examination produced by a professional technologist that requires a higher degree of technical knowledge and skill than ever before to meet today's increasingly high standards.

STEPHEN A. FEIG, MD
Professor of Radiology
Jefferson Medical College
Director, Breast Imaging Center
Thomas Jefferson University Hospital

Preface to the Second Edition

Many of you during the past 4 years have thanked me for writing *Mammography for Radiologic Technologists*. Those words have been my inspiration to write book number two; I have dedicated this edition to you, my peers.

As most of you know, many changes have occurred during these 4 years. Staying on top of the regulations and getting through the first FDA inspection has been a time of trial for all of you. To those of you who have been successful, congratulations. Remember, no other area of radiography is a subject of such scrutiny.

This edition, like the original book, is not designed either (1) to be the final authority in mammography or (2) to redefine the principles of radiography. This book is designed to provide the tools necessary to help you to perform the best possible mammogram for your patient. The technologist who understands the entire imaging chain will be equipped to deal with the most trying situations.

To my friends who have provided input to this edition, a special thank you: Judy Dresbach, RT(R)(M), Lee Kitt, Ph.D., and Laura Meals, RT(R)(M). I also thank those companies whose contributions have helped to make this text complete:

- Agfa Division, Bayer Corporation
- American Cancer Society
- Eastman Kodak Company
- Fischer Imaging Systems
- General Electric Company
- Nuclear Associates
- Philips Medical Systems
- Radiation Measurement Instruments, Inc.
- Siemens Medical Systems, Inc.
- X-rite

I wish to also express appreciation to Cooper Medical Center, Cherry Hill, NJ, which permitted me to use their mammography suite for the photographic session. And to Gettysburg Hospital, Gettysburg, PA, which provided radiographs and continues to support my endeavors.

Last, I wish to thank McGraw-Hill for the opportunity to publish this second edition.

Gini Wentz, RT(R)(M)

Preface to the First Edition

During the last decade, mammography has proved to be a vital diagnostic procedure in improving the quality of a woman's life. The purpose of this book is to provide the mammography technologist with the guidelines for performing quality mammography.

For too long the individuals responsible for performing mammography have been left alone to try to obtain materials for their education. There has been a dearth of "how to" material. I hope that this book will provide information to allow the technologist to go beyond the standard two-view mammogram.

In no way should this book be viewed as the final authority on mammography. It is my goal to provide my fellow mammography technologists with the tools to best perform this lifesaving procedure.

Two individuals have been my inspiration: Stephen A. Feig, MD, and Arthur G. Haus, PhD. Their contribution to mammography has benefited many, and I thank them for their support and encouragement.

It is only fitting to acknowledge with appreciation those individuals and companies who have contributed to this book. Special thanks go to my friends whose support and assistance have contributed to this manuscript: Debra Deibel, RT; Michael Fedyna, RT; Laura Meals, RT; Anne Richards, BART; and Marc Vrielynck.

I also thank those companies whose contributions have helped to make this text complete:

- Agfa–Gevaert N.V.
- Agfa Corporation
- Eastman Kodak Company
- E. I. Du Pont de Nemours & Company, Inc.
- General Electric Company
- Nuclear Associates
- Philips Medical Systems
- Radiation Measurement Instruments, Inc.
- Siemens Medical Systems, Inc.

The support of facilities that have provided reference material and radiographs is also appreciated:

- Medical Center of Central Massachusetts, Worcester, Massachusetts
- The Massachusetts General Hospital, Boston, Massachusetts
- Faulkner-Sagoff Breast Center, Boston, Massachusetts
- Gettysburg Hospital, Gettysburg, Pennsylvania
- Baptist Memorial Hospital, Memphis, Tennessee

Last, I wish to thank my family and friends; without their support this text would not have been possible.

GINI WENTZ, RT

Introduction

The experienced technologist makes mammography appear deceptively effortless. The casual observer can conclude that mammography is simply a matter of purchasing a machine that will take the pictures. It is predictable that such ventures will produce suboptimal results. Mammography technologists are crucial to the production of useful x-ray images of the human breast. Their tasks are far from simple.

No other medical imaging demands the levels of contrast, spatial resolution, and precise positioning required for quality mammography. Mammography is effective in early detection of breast cancers only because of the attention given to the details of producing high-quality images at the limits of available technology.

The interpretation skills of the best radiologist are no match for the suboptimal image. Subtle signs of breast malignancy are detectable only when they are included in the images.

This textbook is intended to be a guide for the novice, a refresher course for the experienced, and a reference for all who are determined to practice high-quality mammography.

WARD PARSONS, MD, RT

Mammography for Radiologic Technologists

1

History of Mammography

The concern for breast disease was documented before W. Roentgen introduced the world to the properties of x-ray in 1895. It has been suggested that Rembrandt's model for Bathsheba (Figure 1.1) had breast cancer. Note the skin dimpling on the lateral aspect of the left breast. This is one clinical indication of breast disease (1).

Between the fifteenth and the seventeenth centuries, European surgeons and physicians fought breast disease with methods that would be considered barbaric by today's standards. Too often, by the time the patient was treated, the tumors were clinically evident and widespread metastasis had occurred. It is felt that surgery often speeded up the metastatic process of the disease.

In 1913, Dr. A. Salomon, a German surgeon from the Surgical University of Berlin, reported the clinical and radiographic findings of the tumored breast. Using glass plates and a conventional x-ray machine, Dr. Salomon evaluated breast specimens. A majority of these findings make up many of the breast cancer classifications referred to today. The patients were often treated surgically; standard practice was a radical mastectomy. It became evident with time, however, that the use of extensive surgery was not improving the patient's survival rate.

In 1930 in the United States, Stafford Warren reported the diagnostic value of performing mammography on the live patient. Unfortunately, because of the inability of facilities to repeat satisfactory image quality, mammography was virtually discontinued.

J. Gershon-Cohen of Philadelphia in 1947 renewed the interest in mammography by correlating the radiographic images with the anatomy and pathology of the breast. Once again, most facilities found it difficult to reproduce images of diagnostic quality.

In the early 1950s, Dr. R. Leborgne of Uruguay reported on the appearances of microcalcifications and their association with certain types of breast cancer. Dr. Leborgne acknowledged the need for perfect technique when performing mammography. He stressed (2):

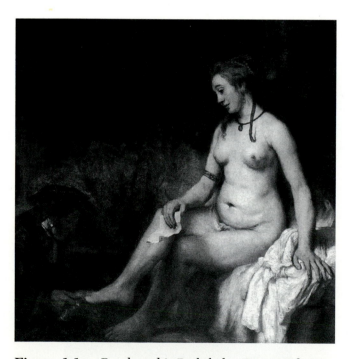

Figure 1.1. Rembrandt's Bathsheba. Reprinted courtesy of the National Museums of France (Musées Nationaux, Paris, France).

- the need to use low-kVp techniques
- the need for collimation by using an extension cone

1

- the value of high-contrast images
- compression

In 1956, Robert Egan, a fellow and staff radiologist at the University of Texas, M.D. Anderson Hospital and Tumor Institute, accepted an assignment to investigate the value of clinical mammography. Four years later, Dr. Egan presented a paper discussing his findings. After many trials testing a variety of factors, Dr. Egan indicated the need to provide consistent quality mammography by (3):

- optimizing the x-ray equipment for radiographing soft tissue, such as the breast
- using dedicated processing and the correct film type
- requiring proper training of technologists and radiologists

To meet those criteria, the following were required (3):

1. Optimizing the x-ray equipment:
   - A conventional diagnostic x-ray unit (Figure 1.2) was used. The filtration was limited to the inherent filtration of the tube (approximately 1 mm of aluminum).
   - The generators and control panels (Figure 1.3) were adapted to accommodate values below

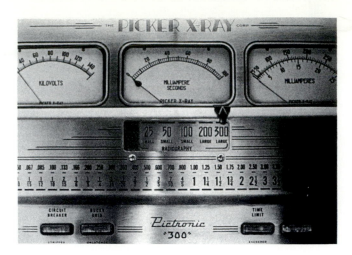

Figure 1.3. A control panel with the exposure factors used for the Egan technique.

30 kVp. The typical exposure factors at this time were 300 mA, 6 s, 26 to 28 kVp. (*Note:* The long exposure factor(s) increased the likelihood of geometric blur or motion.)
   - The focal film distance was kept above 18 in, the extremes being from 22 to 40 in.
   - An extension cylinder cone (Figure 1.2) was used to reduce scatter radiation.
2. Dedicated processing and film:
   - An industrial, extremely fine grain film helped to obtain optimum detail.

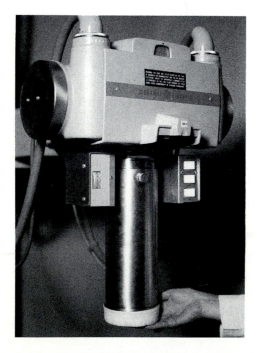

Figure 1.2. Overhead General Electric x-ray tube with cone.

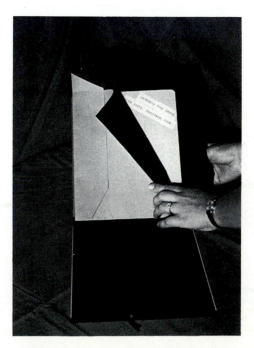

Figure 1.4. Cardboard film holder.

- The film was placed into a cardboard holder (Figure 1.4), preferably with lead backing.
- Manual processing (Figure 1.5) with long developing times, up to 7 1/2 min, was used as well as longer fixing and washing times. The importance of fresh and clean solutions was stressed.

3. Proper training of the radiology staff involved with mammography:
   - Technologists were taught proper positioning and the techniques required to optimize the image quality.
   - Radiologists attended a 1-week course taught by Dr. Egan.

Dr. Egan's finest contribution was his emphasis on the mammography team. Team effort with attention given to all details was imperative to obtain the high image quality necessary for mammography.

Xerography was developed in the late 1930s by Chester F. Carlson. It was not, however, until the 1960s that xerography was employed in medicine. In 1967, at the International Mammography Conference, Dr. J. Wolfe of Detroit presented a paper describing his work with xerography for mammographic applications(4). Shortly after Dr. Wolfe presented his findings, a committee from the American College of Radiology (ACR) asked the Xerox Corporation to continue developing xerography. In 1968 a clinical program was launched by Dr. Wolfe and Dr. J. Martin of Houston. The xerography process proved to be successful in the field of breast imaging.

Xerography requires two units: a conditioner and a processor. First, in the conditioner, a plate is auto-matically prepared for exposure. The preparation depends on a selenium-coated aluminum plate that is a photoconductor. The selenium plate is electrically charged. The plate is placed into a holder, much as film is placed into a cassette (see Chapter 4, Section 2.1). After the plate is exposed to an x-ray beam, a latent image develops on the plate.

In the processor, the plate is removed from the holder. The image becomes visible when exposed to a blue powder of charged particles. The powder image is transferred to a sheet of a plastic-coated paper to produce a mirror image. The paper is heated, and the toner particles become imbedded in the plastic.

The introduction of xerography for mammographic application afforded facilities the ability to further evaluate a patient suspected of having breast cancer. Xeromammography did not require facilities to tailor their x-ray equipment or their darkroom, yet it provided a diagnostic tool. Surgeons benefited by xerography as they were presented with a visual medium to assist them in surgery.

1. Development of Dedicated Mammography Equipment

In the 1960s Professor C. M. Gros of France introduced two additional concepts to the film mammography imaging chain. First, the tungsten (W) target was replaced with a molybdenum (Mo) target tube. Dr. Gros demonstrated that the characteristic radiation resulting from the molybdenum target improved the contrast between the subtle breast architecture: fat, calcification(s), and parenchymal tissue. Second, vigorous compression was applied while exposing the breast. Compression separated the breast tissues to provide a uniform thickness and help eliminate patient motion. Dr. Gros had made major strides in improving image quality, but the skin dose to the patient had increased compared with that of the Egan technique.

Professor Gros and the Compagnie Générale de Radiologie (CGR) in France began developing the first dedicated x-ray unit for mammography. The Senographe® I (Figure 1.6) was introduced at the

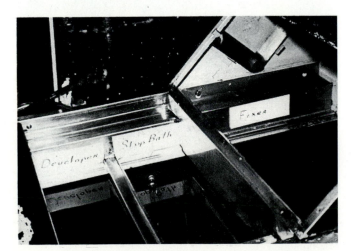

Figure 1.5. Manual processing tanks.

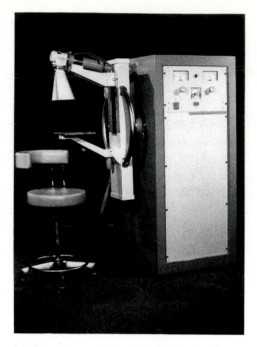

Figure 1.6. Senographe® I. Reprinted courtesy of General Electric Company, Milwaukee, WI.

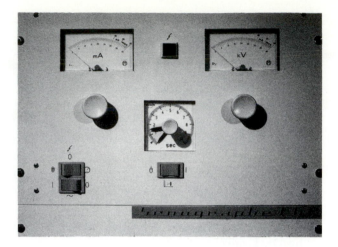

Figure 1.7. Senographe® I: control panel. Reprinted courtesy of General Electric Company, Milwaukee, WI.

1967 Radiological Society of North America (RSNA) meeting and had the following features:

1. X-ray tube stand: A rotating C-arm configuration supported the x-ray tube and a film holder. Patients could be evaluated in the erect or the recumbent position.
2. X-ray tube: The x-ray tube was a water-cooled, stationary molybdenum anode.
3. Window: The window or exit port was a beryllium window, replacing the glass window. A glass window filters out the extremely low energy ("soft") photons required for mammography.
4. Focal spot: The size of the focal spot was improved.
   • a 0.7-mm focal spot replaced the 1.5- to 2.0-mm focal spot
5. Generator-control panel: A dedicated generator was designed for breast imaging. The control panel (Figure 1.7) offered:
   • manual exposure selection
   • up to 40 mA
   • up to 40 kVp
   • up to 10-s time selection
6. Collimation: Interchangeable cones (Figure 1.8) of various shapes and sizes were useful to help minimize scatter radiation.
7. Compression: A piece of plastic was attached to

the bottom of the cone(s) to compress the breast during the exposure.

The disadvantage of this unit was that the compression device was part of the tube-cone assembly. Thus the focal film distance varied from patient to patient and from position to position. Consequently, this variation offset the advantage of the smaller focal spot size. The variable source-to-image distance (SID) caused magnification and/or distortion of the image.

The advantage of this system was the improvement in contrast, resolution, and image quality compared with that of previously performed film mammography.

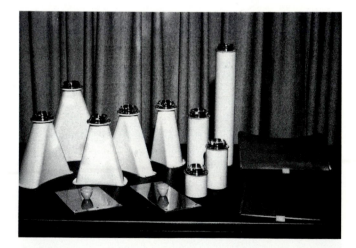

Figure 1.8. Senographe® I: various extension cones. Reprinted courtesy of General Electric Company, Milwaukee, WI.

2. Development of Screen-Film Combinations

In 1972 the Albert Einstein Medical Center in Philadelphia asked E. I. Du Pont de Nemours & Co. in Wilmington, Delaware, to develop a new mammography film. The industrial film type was replaced when Du Pont introduced their LoDose film and LoDose intensifying screens into the market.

Characteristics of the Du Pont LoDose film were as follows:

- wide recording latitude allowing visualization from the chest wall to the nipple
- high resolution permitting visualization of micro-calcifications
- low noise
- low radiation dose to the glandular tissue
- sharpness of the screen-film system, which provided the ability to record the minute structural details. A single screen was used with a single-emulsion film to reduce the "crossover" effect.
- addition of an antihalation backing layer to the film to minimize light reflected from the film base.

This film was coupled with the LoDose intensifying

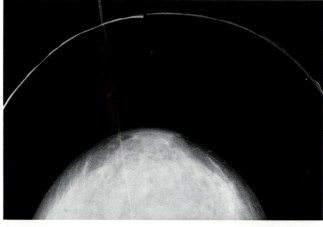

A

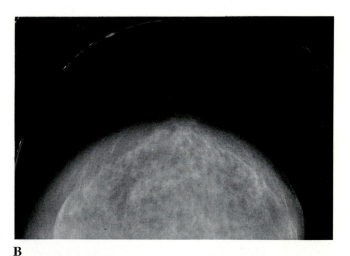

B

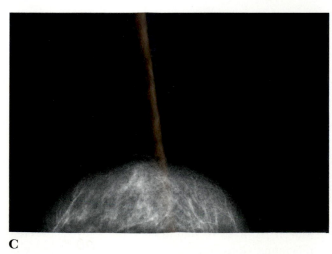

C

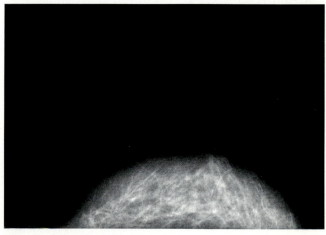

D

Figure 1.9. Improvements in screen-film mammography, performed on one patient.
A. 1978, the Egan technique (300-mA 6-s 28-kVp overhead x-ray tube);
B. 1985, first-generation mammography unit and screen-film system;
C. 1987, second-generation mammography unit and a third-generation screen-film system;
D. Mammography performed in 1990 with all conditions optimized for breast imaging.

screen and was placed in a polyethylene vacuum bag. Introduction of DuPont's LoDose mammography film challenged all the film manufacturers to develop a high-quality film that would reduce the exposure to the patient.

The second-generation mammography screen–film system was introduced in 1976. The introduction of the film holder or dedicated mammography cassette also brought about the introduction of the Min-R screen (see Chapter 4, Section 2.1). The Min-R screen used a gadolinium oxysulfide:tebium phosphor technology. The Min-R screen and film combination was a major contributor to further reduction in exposure. The systems that were available at the time included:

- DuPont LoDose
- Kodak Min-R
- Agfa Mamoray

Other films, such as Sakura C film, were available and were combined with the Min-R screen.

The main benefit of the second generation was that the increase in speed permitted:

- reduction in kVp, again improving the contrast
- reduction in patient motion
- reduction in the amount of heat generated by the tube, prolonging tube life

The Min-R screen-film system was approximately 15 times faster than that of the Kodak Industrex M non-screen film.

In 1978, the third generation of mammography film was introduced. Once again, the system speed reduced exposure to the patient by approximately 50% compared with the second generation. The systems that became available were:

- Kodak Ortho M film and Min-R screen
- NMB film and Min-R screen
- DuPont MRF 31 film with LoDose 2 or LoDose

The screen-film combinations were a single screen and single-emulsion film combination. The increased contrast improved visualization of the small calcification(s).

Initially, it was felt that the third generation was not as good as the second generation (5). The perceived disadvantages were as follows:

- increase in contrast was regarded as a drawback because the nipple, skin line, and subcutaneous fat were "blacked out." A bright light was required to visualize those areas.
- increased system speed created a potential to visualize "quantum mottle" (see Chapter 4, Section 3.2).

Kodak's Ortho M film was faster than Min-R film and was therefore an excellent choice for magnification studies or grid work. Other advantages of this system were as follows:

- reduction in exposure time reduced patient motion
- increased speed permitted greater flexibility in exposure factors

The introduction of the new screen-film combinations and dedicated mammography equipment resulted in a reduction in patient dose that at one time was felt to be unattainable. Exposure factors had been reduced drastically, and image quality had not suffered. As seen in Figure 1.9, the advancements made in screen-film mammography over the past 20 years have been impressive.

Acknowledgment: I would like to thank Russell Holland for his assistance and valuable input on the section "Development of Screen-Film Combinations."

References

1. Degenshein GA, Coccarelli F. The history of breast cancer surgery. Breast Dis 1977;3:34.
2. Leborgne R. Diagnosis of tumors of the breast by simple Roentgenographe: Calcifications in carcinomas. Roentgenol Radium Ther 1951;65(1):1–11.
3. Egan RL. Breast Imaging, 3rd ed. Baltimore: University Park Press; 1984:1–5.
4. Martin JE. Atlas of Mammography: Histologic Mammographic Correlations. 2nd ed. Baltimore: Williams & Wilkins; 1988:55.
5. Sickles EA. Efforts to lower dose and maximize diagnostic accuracy. Presented at the 20th National Breast Conference on Breast Cancer; March 15, 1982; New Orleans.

2

Overview of Breast Imaging

Mammography, the most effective noninvasive means available for examining the breast, is usually associated with the search for breast cancers, although most patients examined with mammography either are normal or have benign disease.

That which we call *breast cancer* is a collection of diseases with different cellular characteristics, growth rates, and metastatic tendencies. In the treatment of breast cancers, patient response varies from rapid demise to long-term survival. Breast cancers are not preventable with current technology. Although early detection does not guarantee a favorable outcome, extensive scientific evidence indicates that early detection and appropriate treatment of breast cancers significantly reduce the mortality from this family of diseases.

Mammography is the most sensitive and accurate method known for detecting occult breast cancer. No test for breast cancer is perfect. Mammography is imperfect in a predictable fashion. It is less effective when used to examine the radiographically dense glandular breast, in which isodense lesions can be concealed.

Mammography is not always diagnostically specific. Benign and malignant processes can cause similar, sometimes identical mammographic changes. Distinguishing one from the other with imaging alone is not always possible. Biopsy is usually needed to make the distinction. Less than half of all mammographically recommended breast biopsies reveal ma-

lignant disease. Most biopsies identify benign breast diseases that have caused suspicious alterations of the normal mammographic image.

Mammography fails to detect some breast cancers. Some failures result from technical inadequacies or errors of perception or interpretation. Others occur because breast carcinomas do not always produce a recognizable change in the mammographic image. Mammography complements but cannot replace regular physical examination and breast self-examination (BSE). Palpable cancers are not always visible. Visible cancers are not always palpable.

The benefits of properly performed and interpreted mammography have been demonstrated in several studies. Randomized controlled studies have included groups of women divided into two populations with similar characteristics. The study groups were invited to mammographic screening; the control groups were not. The breast cancer death rates for the invited study groups are typically lower than the rates for the unscreened control groups.

In the early 1960s, the Health Insurance Plan of New York began a study of 62,000 women over age 40, offering annual mammographic screening to half of the women for 4 years (HIP Study) (1). Although just over half of the women in the study group attended all four of the screens, their group obtained a more than 30% reduction in breast cancer mortality compared with the control group. Similar results were obtained in a study of 15,000 women in Utrecht,

7

the Netherlands (2). Another Dutch study in the city of Nijmegen resulted in an almost 50% mortality reduction in a controlled study of 30,000 women (3).

In the 1970s, a nationwide study known as the Breast Cancer Detection Demonstration Project (BCDDP) involved 28 sites and a total of 280,000 women in the United States (4). The BCDDP concluded that mammography can detect breast cancer at an earlier stage than physical examination, that a high proportion of these cancers were found while still localized to the breast, and that mortality was reduced more than 40% compared with the unscreened population.

The Swedish Two County Trial, started in 1977 with over 130,000 women, has resulted in a 30% reduction in breast cancer mortality for the group invited to screening (5).

In the United States, the average woman has about 1 chance in 8 of developing breast cancer during her lifetime. Approximately 45,000 women in the United States are expected to die from breast cancer in 1996. A mammography screening program with a 30% mortality reduction could theoretically prevent 13,000 breast cancer deaths per year.

Breast cancer statistics derived from population studies are of limited value in application to individuals. All women are at risk for developing breast cancer (absolute risk). The risk increases with age (Figure 2.1). We cannot determine which woman will or will not develop breast cancer.

Some groups of the female population are at greater or lesser risk than others because of factors other than gender and age (relative risk). Hormonal status, pregnancy and lactation, and family or personal history of breast disease are considered in estimating risk, but none of these can be used to make accurate individual predictions. Most breast malignancies occur in women who have none of the commonly acknowledged risk factors. Known risk factors do not provide a basis for selective screening.

The two applications of mammography are *screening* and *diagnosis*. The purpose of screening is to search for breast cancer in asymptomatic women who are expected to be without disease. Women who have symptoms or abnormal physical findings should be directed to diagnostic study.

Are there any women who can or should be excluded from screening? This question can be addressed but not definitively answered. Desirable results (benefits) usually come at some cost (risk). We know that the benefit of screening mammography is early detection of breast cancer with improved likelihood of cure.

Radiation exposure to women under age 35 could theoretically result in an increase in the incidence of breast cancer. Since patients less than 35 years old develop fewer breast cancers than older patients and because these younger women might be more sensitive to the effects of radiation, they are usually not included in mammographic screening programs. Males are not screened because the rarity of breast malignancy in asymptomatic men makes the procedure impractical.

Screening guidelines exclude pregnant and lactating patients to avoid potential errors in examining the physiologically altered, mammographically dense breast.

Safe and effective techniques are available for mammographic study of patients with breast implants. These patients are technically challenging, but they can benefit from properly performed screening studies.

The American Cancer Society (ACS) and the American College of Radiology (ACR) have developed guidelines for mammographic screening of asymptomatic women:

- age 35–40: baseline mammogram
- age 40–49: mammograms at 1- to 2-year intervals
- age 50: annual mammograms

These screening guidelines are endorsed by many but not all professional medical organizations. Patient selection criteria for mammographic screening are controversial. The scientific community accepts postmenopausal screening mammography as effective for

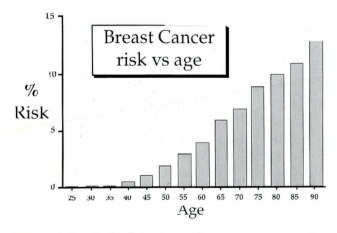

Figure 2.1. Risk of developing breast cancer according to age.

the reduction of breast cancer mortality. Evidence of effectiveness in premenopausal patients is abundant. Economic and political considerations have further complicated the situation (6–9).

With properly performed screening, one can detect occult breast cancers by identifying patients with suspicious findings that require biopsy. Of these biopsies, half or more will indicate benign disease.

After a few years of screening, good baseline studies will have been established for the population. Sensitivity in detection of malignancies increases, since only mammographic changes will require evaluation. We expect to find fewer lesions that require biopsy, but a greater portion of these will be malignant.

Regular periodic screening reduces the number of biopsies necessary to find most of the malignancies. A few patients will discover breast cancers between screenings. Others will develop malignancies that are not detectable with current imaging techniques. These might be palpable lesions or neoplasms that cause nipple discharge. Occasionally, a patient will present with enlarged lymph nodes or widespread metastatic disease with no mammographically visible breast lesion.

Screening should be used only to detect abnormalities requiring further study. Breast biopsy should not be recommended on the basis of a screening mammogram unless the abnormality is unequivocal. Many breast lesions are multifocal. Detailed imaging workup can characterize suspicious lesions and detect additional disease not apparent on standard images. Intervention before proper diagnostic workup can lead to unnecessary biopsies or inadequate excisions.

Diagnostic imaging of the breast is used in the workup of screening abnormalities, imaging of the symptomatic patient, or analysis of abnormal physical findings, where it can solve problems. Magnification, spot compression, angulation techniques, and ancillary modalities—(ultrasound, fine needle aspiration (FNA), core biopsy, ductography, pneumocystography)—are available to increase specificity and define the extent of disease.

Patients with palpable breast neoplasms should be examined to characterize the palpable lesion and to search for occult lesions in both breasts. Occasionally, the palpable mass is benign and occult cancer exists in the same and/or opposite breast.

Ultrasound plays an important role in the diagnosis of breast disease. It accurately distinguishes cystic from solid lesions (matrix determination) and helps to distinguish benign from malignant solid tissues. Ultrasound is an excellent guide for many interventional procedures. Breast ultrasound is not yet an adequate screening procedure.

Fine needle aspiration with cytologic examination or core biopsy with histologic examination are accurate, minimally invasive diagnostic procedures. With stereotactic or ultrasound guidance, preoperative tissue diagnosis can reduce the need for surgery in benign disease or aid in treatment planning when the findings are malignant.

Ductography is used to identify intraductal lesions in patients who have single-duct nipple discharge. Ductography can determine whether lesions are single or multiple and assist in their localization. Injection of an indicator dye (methylene blue) into the abnormal duct can guide surgical dissection.

Pneumocystography is an air contrast study obtained by replacing aspirated cyst fluid with air and performing a mammogram, usually with magnification. It is useful when ultrasound detects an atypical cyst, intracystic lesion, or mural nodule; when a cyst aspirate is bloody; and when rapidly recurring cysts are encountered.

Periodic studies of the postlumpectomy/postirradiation breast are important because these patients have a higher risk of developing cancer in the opposite breast or recurrence at the surgical site. New baseline mammography is usually performed 3 to 6 months after treatment, then at 6-month intervals for 3 years. Once stability has been reestablished, annual studies are recommended. Imaging of mastectomy sites can detect some local recurrences that are not clinically apparent, but this practice is generally not cost-effective.

Mammography is encouraged for screening-age patients *prior* to augmentation or reduction mammoplasty. An occult lesion hidden by an implant or by postoperative architectural change could result in delayed diagnosis.

Preoperative wire localization of occult lesions is essential in the management of the patient with suspected breast cancer. Image-guided biopsies are usually faster, less deforming, and more accurate. Specimen radiography is essential for confirmation of accurate and complete excision of pathology.

Computed tomography (CT), magnetic resonance imaging (MRI), and positron emission tomography (PET) are occasionally useful to evaluate of unusual lesions, to resolve difficult localization problems, and to facilitate staging. Magnetic resonance imaging offers some advantages in study of breast implants. These modalities are not practical for routine breast evaluation.

Small field-of-view digital mammography is effective in stereotactic applications and for some localizations. Large-field digital systems are under development. Digital image enhancement techniques, dose reduction, image storage/retrieval/transmission improvements, and computer-aided diagnosis are anticipated benefits of technological progress.

Breast imaging has much to offer in the detection, diagnosis, and management of breast diseases. It is no longer just mammography.

References

1. Strax P, Venet L, Shapiro S. Value of mammography in reduction of mortality from breast cancer in mass screening. AJR 1973;117:686–689.
2. Collette HJA, Day NE, Rombach JJ, deWaard F. Evaluation of screening for breast cancer in a non-randomized study (The DOM Project) by means of case control study. Lancet 1984;1:1224–1226.
3. Verbeek, ALM, Hendriks JHCL, Holland R, et al. Reduction of breast cancer mortality through mass screening with modern mammography: First results of the Nijmegen Project 1975–1981. Lancet 1984;1:1222–1224.
4. Seidman H, Gelb S, Silverberg E, et al. Survival experience in the breast cancer detection demonstration project. CA 1987;37:258–290.
5. Tabar L, Fagerberg G, Duffy SW, Day NE, Gad A, Grontoft O. Update of the Swedish two-county program of mammographic screening for breast cancer. Radiol Clin North Am 1992;30:187–210.
6. Curpen BN, Sickles EA, Sillitto RA, et al. The comparative value of mammographic screening for women 40–49 years old versus women 50–64 years old. AJR 1995;164:1099–1103.
7. Feig S. Decreased breast cancer mortality through mammographic screening: Results of clinical trials. Radiology 1988;167:659–665.
8. Mettlin C, Smart CR, Breast cancer detection guidelines for women aged 40–49 years: Rationale for the American Cancer Society Reaffirmation of Recommendations. CA 1994;44:248–255.
9. Sickles EA. American College of Radiology statement on screening mammography for women 40–49. ACR Bull 1993; 4–93.

3

Anatomy and Physiology of the Breast

1. The Normal Breast

An understanding of breast anatomy is essential to the performance of high-quality mammography. Technologists can apply their knowledge of anatomy to properly position and compress the breast so that as much tissue as possible is imaged without harm to the patient. The finest equipment and flawless processing cannot compensate for substandard positioning.

2. External Anatomy

The adult female breasts are a pair of approximately symmetrical hemispheric tissue mounds on the anterior chest wall between the skin and the pectoral muscles. The breasts extend vertically from the second rib to the sixth and horizontally from the sternal edge to the midaxillary line, usually with extension toward the axilla (Figure 3.1A).

Normal breasts vary in size and contour, from flattened domes to conical, spherical, or pendulous forms. The weight and size of the breasts change with age, generally increasing after puberty, increasing further with pregnancy and lactation, and decreasing with the atrophy of aging. The breasts are enclosed in thin skin that contains hair follicles, sebaceous glands, and sweat glands.

The centrally located areola is a circular pigmented area of skin measuring from about 2 to 6 cm in diameter. The elevations around the perimeter of the areola are Morgagni's tubercles, formed by the openings of the ducts of Montgomery's glands.

The nipple, located in the center of the areola, is usually a protuberance of 5 to 10 mm in diameter. It contains 5 to 10 openings of the major ducts converging from the branching system of ducts that drain the milk-producing glandular lobes of the breast. Normal nipples can be flattened or inverted.

3. Internal Anatomy

The breast is loosely attached to the fascia covering the pectoralis major muscle. This allows the breast to move over the chest wall. The attachments are most restrictive superiorly and medially, an important feature to remember when positioning the breast for a mammogram. The lateral border of the breast and the inframammary fold are the most mobile portions. Compression of the breast is most effective and most comfortable when applied in the mobile areas.

Beneath the skin of the breast is a layer of superficial fascia continuous with a layer of deep fascia. These fascial layers form an envelope that contains

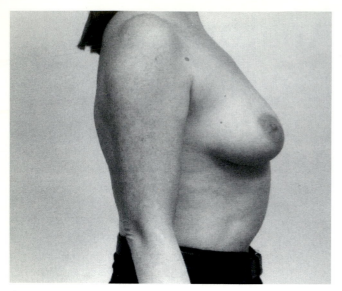

A

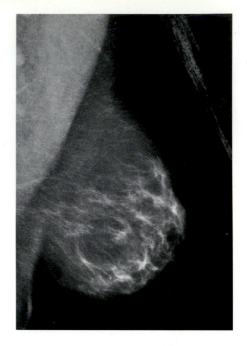

B

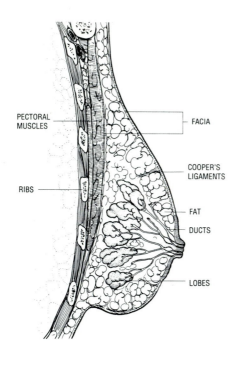

PECTORAL MUSCLES

FACIA

RIBS

COOPER'S LIGAMENTS

FAT

DUCTS

LOBES

C

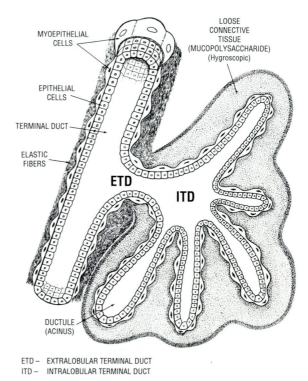

MYOEPITHELIAL CELLS

LOOSE CONNECTIVE TISSUE (MUCOPOLYSACCHARIDE) (Hygroscopic)

EPITHELIAL CELLS

TERMINAL DUCT

ELASTIC FIBERS

ETD

ITD

DUCTULE (ACINUS)

ETD – EXTRALOBULAR TERMINAL DUCT
ITD – INTRALOBULAR TERMINAL DUCT

D

Figure 3.1. Anatomy of the female breast. **A.** Patient positioned in the lateral projection. **B.** Mediolateral oblique projection. **C.** Lateral view of the female breast. **D.** Microscopic anatomy of the terminal duct lobular unit.

all of the mammary tissues. This envelope rests on loose fatty tissue in the retromammary space anterior to the pectoralis major muscle (Figure 3.1C).

Breast tissues are of three major types: (1) fibrous, (2) glandular or secretory, and (3) adipose or fatty. The fatty tissues are radiolucent, resulting in areas of higher optical density on the mammogram. The fibrous and glandular tissues are usually de-

scribed together as fibroglandular densities. These result in areas of lower optical density on the mammogram (Figure 3.1B).

The radiographic contrast or difference in density of these two tissue groups allows us to image the breast. The density differences are small. A high-contrast mammographic imaging system is necessary to make breast anatomy visible.

The breasts are supported and given shape by a network of fibrous and elastic bands known as Cooper's ligaments. These extend from the deep skin layer through the mammary tissues to the deep fascia. Cooper's ligaments are visible on the normal mammogram as thin, gently curving lines. They can be shortened or straightened by the fibrosis associated with breast cancer, causing skin retraction or localized architectural distortion. High-resolution mammographic technique is necessary for adequate visualization to these structures.

Beneath the skin and superficial fascia is a layer of adipose tissue about 1 to 2 cm thick. Behind this layer is the mammary stroma, a mixture of supportive connective tissue, fat, blood vessels, lymphatic channels, ducts, and the lobes of glandular tissues.

The relative amounts of fat and glandular tissue vary with age, body weight, and heredity. Generally, glandular tissues predominate in the young woman, adipose tissues in the older patient; but this is not a consistent relationship. Breasts that contain large amounts of glandular tissue and little fat are more difficult to image because of the low subject contrast. The only reliable, noninvasive means of determining the ratio of fat to glandular tissue is to obtain a quality mammogram.

The glandular tissues are arranged in 10 to 15 overlapping lobes, each with a collecting duct that leads to the nipple. Most of the glandular tissue is found in the central portion of the breast and in the upper outer quadrant, extending toward the axilla. Since breast cancers arise from glandular tissue, mammographic positioning must include as much glandular tissue as possible on the images.

4. Vascular and Lymphatic Anatomy

The blood supply to the breasts comes from the internal mammary and lateral thoracic arteries. Arterial branches that develop calcifications are well displayed on high-contrast, high-resolution mammograms. Sharp images are important to avoid mistaking vascular calcifications for calcifications of malignant disease.

Normal lymphatic channels in the breast are too small to visualize. These channels can enlarge to become important identifying elements of certain disease states. Normal axillary and intramammary lymph nodes are commonly visible on properly positioned mammograms. The typical lymph node is an ovoid structure with a lucent center, or hilum. Normal nodes can be several centimeters in length. Enlarged nodes or nodes with solid centers can indicate either benign or malignant disease.

5. Microscopic Anatomy

Each of the glandular lobes is divided into lobules. The lobule and its duct form the basic histopathologic unit of the breast, the terminal ductal lobular unit (TDLU). Most benign and malignant lesions of the breast originate in the TDLU. In high quality mammographic images, the TDLUs are displayed as overlapping densities 1 to 2 mm in diameter.

The lobule is composed of an intralobular terminal duct and multiple sac-like ductules lined with a single layer of epithelial cells and a peripheral layer of myoepithelial cells. The cellular layers are separated from the other breast tissues by a boundary layer known as the basement membrane. The lobule and intralobular terminal duct components of the TDLU are embedded in loose connective tissue. The extralobular terminal ducts have the same two cellular layers plus periductal elastic fibers (Figure 3.2A&B).

6. Normal Physiology

During lactation, the TDLUs increase in size and number. The epithelial cells secrete milk. Hormonal stimulation causes contraction of the myoepithelial cells, expressing milk into the main lactiferous ducts toward the nipple. After lactation ceases, the TDLUs shrink, and many disappear. After menopause, more lobules disappear and the small ducts become atrophic. The breast often becomes entirely replaced by fatty tissue.

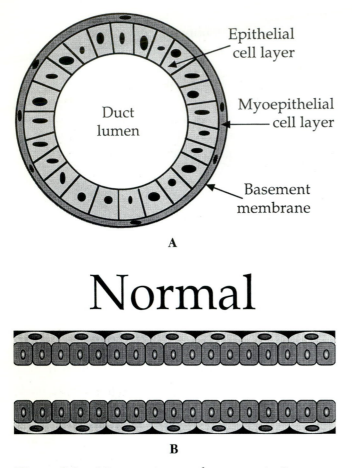

Normal

Figure 3.2. Microscopic normal anatomy. **A.** Cross section of the normal duct. **B.** Longitudinal section of the normal duct.

7. The Abnormal Breast

Knowledge of the morphology of breast diseases is essential to understanding their mammographic and ultrasound appearances. Abnormalities of the breast are traditionally separated into the categories of benign and malignant. The breasts have a limited range of responses to disease. Normal tissues can be replaced or displaced by neoplasm. Benign and malignant entities can cause similar morphological changes. Deciding between the two can be difficult, requiring thorough workup techniques, ancillary imaging modalities, and, ultimately, tissue sampling.

8. Breast Masses

The most common mammographic abnormality is the mass. A mass is a three-dimensional tissue structure sufficiently different from its surroundings to become visible as a contrasting element in the mammographic image. Some masses are palpable, some are detectable with ultrasound. Masses vary in contour from sharply defined and spherical through degrees of lobulation and marginal irregularity to the classic spiculated forms of invasive malignancy.

Masses are categorized by their matrix characteristics as either cystic or solid structures. Ultrasound is the most specific noninvasive technique available for matrix determination. The mammographic image is not reliable for this purpose. The most common benign breast masses are cysts and fibroadenomas.

9. Cysts

Cysts are distended TDLUs. Fluid accumulates in the acini, distending the units up to several centimeters in diameter. This can be the result of overproduction of fluid or of an obstruction to the normal flow and resorption of fluid. The cellular lining of the typical cyst is flattened, nonsecretory epithelium. The apocrine variety of cyst maintains a tall columnar epithelial lining in which the cells are actively secretory. Cysts on ultrasound examination are anechoic structures with sharply defined margins and distal acoustic enhancement.

Simple cysts are fluid-filled, thin-walled cavities. Complex cysts have irregularities such as wall thickening, intracystic debris, septations, or intracystic masses that can be benign or malignant.

10. Solid Masses

The most common benign, solid, circular, or oval mass in the breast is the fibroadenoma. As the name implies, this mass contains fibrous and adenomatous or glandular elements. A proliferation of fibrous tissue encases and attenuates the trapped glandular elements of the TDLUs. Older, degenerating fibroadenomas often develop internal calcifications that resemble popcorn on the mammogram. The ultrasound image of the fibroadenoma is that of a solid, uniform, hypoechoic nodule with sharply defined margins and distal acoustic enhancement.

Any breast mass could be a malignancy; however, irregular and spiculated solid masses are more likely to be malignant than are the homogeneous, circumscribed, circular masses. The classic invasive cancer on a mammogram is a stellate or starburst-shaped structure with spicules of various lengths.

In-situ

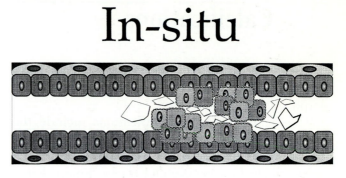

Figure 3.3. Microscopic anatomy. Longitudinal section of ductal carcinoma in situ.

11. Proliferative Abnormalities

The common breast lesions originate in and around the TDLUs. The cells lining the terminal ducts are subject to various degrees of abnormal growth and proliferation described as hyperplasia, atypia, carcinoma in situ, and invasive carcinoma. The transitions from one category to the next are often gradual and difficult to define.

Hyperplasia is an increase in the size and number of otherwise normal epithelial cells. *Atypia* is an abnormal form of hyperplasia in which the cells have distorted morphology and arrangement but no malignant features. *Malignant breast lesions* are in situ and invasive cancers.

13. Invasive Malignancies

Malignant cells that break through the basement membrane become an invasive cancer (Figure 3.4). The invading cells have access to the vascular and lymphatic channels of the breast, through which they can spread to other organs as metastatic disease. Invasive breast malignancies are categorized by pathologists as the common type, NOS (*not otherwise specified*), or as one of many special forms. The common feature of invasive malignancies is the production of a mass or localized architectural distortion.

12. In Situ Malignancies

Carcinoma in situ [(CIS), ductal carcinoma in situ (DCIS), intraductal carcinoma, noninvasive carcinoma; (Figure 3.3)] is a proliferation of cancerous epithelial cells lining the duct, sometimes extending into and even filling the lumen but not crossing the basement membrane. Some forms of carcinoma in situ fill the ducts with necrotic debris and pleomorphic calcifications.

Invasive

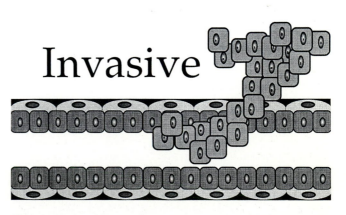

Figure 3.4. Microscopic anatomy. Longitudinal section of invasive ductal carcinoma.

14. Calcifications

Breast calcifications are divided into benign, indeterminate, and malignant categories based on their morphology and distribution.

Classic benign-type calcifications include the round, hollow forms seen in the skin or in areas of fat necrosis. Vascular calcifications follow arterial walls, usually forming parallel tracks. Fine calcium precipitates in fluid will settle to the bottoms of cysts, giving the fluid/mineral levels visible on horizontal beam images— the "teacup" phenomenon. Secretory-type calcifications are solidified secretions that are shaped like the usually large, smooth, and cylindrical ducts in which they are molded. Involutional calcifications are uniform punctate round forms scattered throughout the breast, trapped in shrunken TDLUs.

The calcifications associated with the necrotic cells of carcinoma in situ are *pleomorphic* (meaning "many forms") and ductally oriented. Pleomorphic calcifications are the only reliable mammographic evidence of noninvasive microscopic breast malignancy. They occasionally occur in atypical hyperplasia and sclerosing adenosis, causing differential diagnostic problems for the mammographer. Our best tool for analysis of calcification is high-resolution microfocus magnification mammography.

15. Summary

The common abnormalities of the breast include masses and calcifications. The common benign breast masses are cysts and fibroadenomas. Breast malignancies can be in situ, detected as mammographic microcalcifications, or invasive types that form irregular masses. An understanding of these abnormalities provides the foundation for basic mammographic analysis.

4

The Image

The mammographic image is the result of a photographic process.

1. The dedicated mammography x-ray unit generates an x-ray beam. The beam passes through the breast. A portion of the x-ray beam is absorbed by the breast. The remaining x-ray beam travels until it is recorded by the film-screen image receptor.
2. The latent image, recorded in the emulsion of the exposed film, becomes visible during the development process. The latent image becomes permanent through the chemical actions in the fixer, wash, and finally the drying process.
3. The parameters of development are predetermined to give the desired image density and contrast in a specific time (1,2).

Breast imaging, more than any other diagnostic radiographic procedure, requires technical precision. Proper imaging parameters are essential to evaluate the minute structures within the breast. In this chapter, factors that contribute to providing a high-quality image are discussed, including dedicated mammography equipment, dedicated image receptor (film, cassette, and screen), processing conditions, and darkroom environment. The goal here is not to redefine the concepts of radiography but only to point out those factors that are unique to mammography.

1. Dedicated Mammography Equipment

During the last decade, interest in screening mammography has increased. Many equipment companies have developed dedicated mammography units (Figure 4.1). Prominent mammographers and medical physicists as well as numerous regulatory bodies have established criteria for the dedicated mammography equipment. In this section, those criteria are discussed.

1.1. Tube Stand

The tube stand is designed with a swiveling C-arm type of configuration. The C arm has the x-ray tube mounted in an optimized geometric relationship to the platform that holds the image receptor (film holder). This C-arm type of configuration permits positioning of the patient erect (sitting or standing) or recumbent. The ability to have the patient stand during the procedure often results in an increase in the number of patient procedures performed each day.

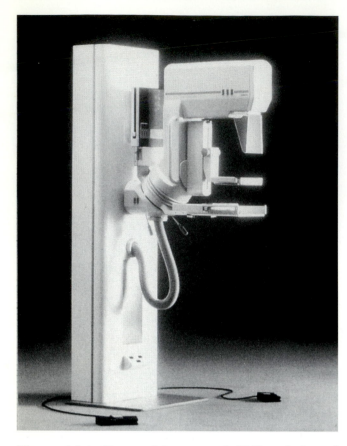

Figure 4.1. Siemens Mammomat® 3000, a dedicated mammography machine. Reprinted courtesy of Siemens Medical Systems, Inc., Iselin, NJ.

1.2. X-Ray Tube Design

It is imperative to have an x-ray tube designed for mammography. Recent improvements in the design of x-ray tubes have permitted an increase in output, as these tubes can withstand higher heat loads. As the patient volume in most mammography departments is increasing, the ability of an x-ray tube to withstand additional exposures facilitates the handling of the increased patient volume.

Radiography of soft tissue requires special target materials and filtration. Today the target materials used for mammography are molybdenum, rhodium, or tungsten. The high-quality radiation from these targets is necessary for displaying the subtle contrast differences of the breast (Figure 4.2).

It is imperative that the correct filtration be coupled with the correct target material. The proper combination provides the low-energy or "soft" x-ray beam needed. The most common target and filtra-

tion combination available is the molybdenum target with 0.03-mm molybdenum filtration. Other target and filtration combinations available are:

- molybdenum target with 0.03-mm molybdenum filtration
- rhodium target with 0.025-mm rhodium filtration. (This target-filtration combination improves penetration of very dense or thick breasts but generally results in lower contrast—particularly for small, fatty breasts.)
- specialized tungsten target with the appropriate K edge filters: molybdenum, rhodium, yttrium, or aluminum (These filters can improve penetrating and reduce mean glandular dose in the dense breast.)

Tungsten and rhodium targets coupled with various filters will alter the spectrum of the x-ray beam. Historically, altering kVp was the only method of altering the beam quality, especially for the dense breast tissue type. The multiple target(s) and/or filtration combinations permit more flexibility to address specific tissue-type requirements. Several manufacturers have introduced dual anode-filtration combinations, for example:

- molybdenum and tungsten target with molybdenum and rhodium filtration
- molybdenum and rhodium target with molybdenum and rhodium filtration

These variable target and filter combinations can improve penetration and reduce mean glandular dose in the dense breast. The objective is to provide the highest image quality with the lowest dose. However, when the adipose breast is radiographed, there may be a slight loss in contrast.

The material used for the exit port or the window is equally important. Conventional x-ray tubes have a glass window that hardens the beam. In mammography, a glass window severely diminishes contrast. Beryllium (Be) permits the soft characteristic radiation to emerge from the x-ray tube, thereby enhancing subject contrast.

The intensity on the anode side is less than that on the cathode side. This variation of the x-ray beam intensity is known as the *heel effect*. The higher cathode-side output of the x-ray tube is always directed to the base of the breast, where the thickness is the greatest.

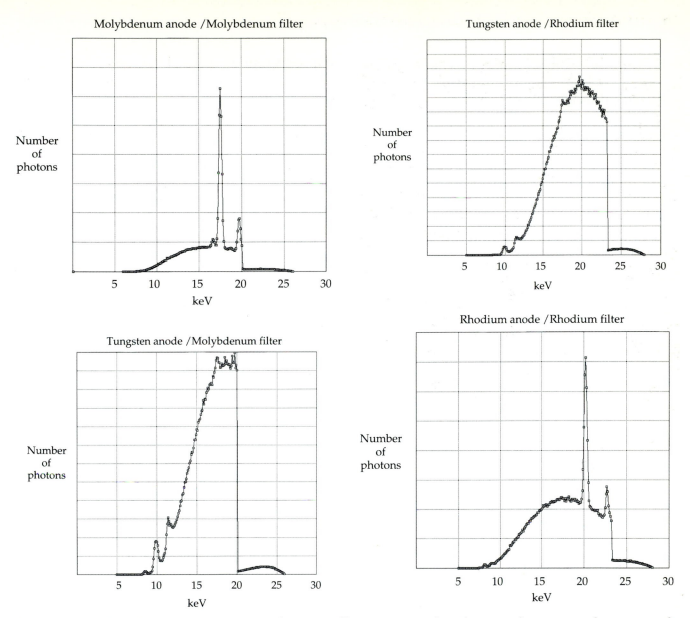

Figure 4.2. Typical x-ray emission spectra for screen-film mammography. These graphs compare the spectra of a molybdenum (Mo) target and molybdenum (Mo) filter, a tungsten (W) target and Mo filter, tungsten target and rhodium (Rh) filter, and a rhodium target and rhodium filter. Data courtesy of Stefan Thunberg.

1.3. Focal Spot

The focal spot is the area of the target from which the x-ray beam is emitted. The focal spot sizes utilized today are smaller than those of the earlier generation. Equipment with a dual focal spot is available. The larger focal spot is used for routine or contact work and the smaller focal spot is used for magnification. The recommended focal spot sizes employed in mammography are:

- 0.4 mm or smaller for routine work (*Note:* 0.3 mm is preferred)
- 0.15 mm or smaller for magnification work

The nominal focal spot size for the large focal spot must be less than or equal to 0.6 mm. Regulations permit the actual or nominal focal spot size to be 50% larger than the actual focal spot stated in the manufacturer's documentation. (Some regulations require limiting spatial resolution requirements be met.) The limiting spatial resolution should be a 13-line pair (l/pr) parallel to the anode-cathode axis by an 11-l/pr perpendicular to the anode-cathode axis. In the small focal spot mode, the resolutions should be no lower than stated: 13- by 11-l/pr.

The size and shape of the focal spot are determined by several factors (3,4):

- size and shape of the electron beam hitting the anode
- design and relationship of the filament coil to the focusing cup
- angle of the anode

Two terms always used when discussing the focal spot are defined as follows (Figure 4.3):

1. The *actual focal spot* is the area on the anode that is bombarded by the electrons discharged from the filament.
2. The *effective focal spot* is the x-ray beam projected toward the patient and the film.

The size of the focal spot is important in mammography, especially when magnification views are made. Resolution and sharpness are directly affected by the focal spot size, the source-to-image distance (SID), and the relationship between the two (5–8). The advantage of an extremely small focal spot is lost if the SID is too short (see Section 1.4).

1.4. Source-to-Image Distance

The SID must be independent of the compression device. Some manufacturers offer the option of a variable SID. This feature is often used when doing stereotactic work. The SID will vary from 50 to 80 cm. The recommended SID is 60 or 65 cm, especially when the focal spot sizes are 0.4 mm or smaller. The goal is to have the smallest focal spot with the longest SID with minimum exposure to the patient (5–7).

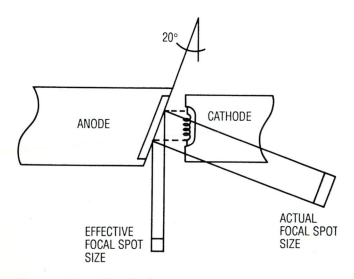

20°

ANODE   CATHODE

EFFECTIVE FOCAL SPOT SIZE

ACTUAL FOCAL SPOT SIZE

Figure 4.3. The focal spot.

1.5. Object-to-Film Distance

Object-to-film distance must be as small as possible. Raising the breast away from the image receptor will result in magnification of the breast as well as loss of resolution. The only time the breast should be positioned away from the receptor is while microfocus magnification views are performed. This is discussed in more detail in Section 1.13.

1.6. Generator Types

The generator types available in mammography are single-phase, three-phase, high-frequency, and constant-potential. Most new units have high-frequency or constant-potential generators, which provide a high-voltage wave form with less than 10% ripple.

The high-frequency and constant-potential generators provide the most homogeneous x-ray beam. A three-phase 12-pulse generator has a minimal ripple factor (approximately 3%) that will affect image quality. The advantage of a three-phase generator is the ability to increase the tube capacity or the mA output. This results in a lower exposure time, reducing patient motion and image blurriness. A conventional single-phase unit produces low-intensity radiation during exposure. The result is longer exposure time with the possibility of patient motion. A single-phase power source may be used with a high-frequency generator, which, like the three-phase generator, increases tube capacity, or mA output. *Note:* The quality of radiation does not change with the different generators: the quantity of radiation is most important (we want the voltage to be close to 100% as possible).

A technologist has no control over the generator design of the equipment type selected. However, the generator type will affect the exposure factors selected. The manufacturers should be consulted for their recommendations.

1.7. kVp Range

The mammography equipment must have the optimum kVp selection required to obtain high subject contrast. Most equipment has the option to select from 20 to 49 kVp in 1-kVp increments. The recommended kVp ranges are dependent upon the target and filtration material(s) utilized.

- molybdenum target tube: from 24 to 30 kVp
- rhodium target tube from 26 to 32 kVp
- tungsten target tube: from 22 to 26 kVp

The kVp used will also depend on radiologist preference, equipment calibration, manufacturer's recommendations, equipment design, characteristic(s) of the screen-film combination, processing, patient breast size and thickness, and so forth (see Chapter 6, "Techniques in Screen-Film Mammography").

1.8. mA Output

Improvements in the x-ray tubes and generators have resulted in an increase in the mA output. The higher mA output permits patient exposure times to be reduced. Shorter exposure times assist in eliminating patient motion. Those tubes with two focal spots have variable mA output. The mA output of the small focal spot is considerably lower than that of the large focal spot. The output of the focal spots will vary according to tube design and generator type. It is preferred that the mA output be as follows:

- large focal spot: 100 mA or greater
- small focal spot: 15 mA or greater

More importantly, at 28 kVp, the radiation output at the entrance surface of the breast should be at least 800 mR/s, and this output should be sustained for at least 3 s. The disadvantages of a lower mA output include (7,8):

- longer exposure times
- increased potential for patient motion
- increased potential for reciprocity failure to occur

Exposures longer than 1 to 2 s may result in the loss of film speed (Section 2.3).

1.9. Automatic Exposure Control (Phototiming)

With modern high-contrast mammographic imaging systems, automatic exposure control (AEC) is essential. An AEC is a device that controls the length of exposure to result in the desired image density. An AEC helps to eliminate the guesswork in determining the proper exposure factors for each patient. Currently, there are three types of AECs: the photomultiplier, the ionization chamber, and solid state.

The users should check with the manufacturer to determine the type of AEC installed into their equipment.

It is important to have the AEC adjusted for the cassette, the screen-film combination, and the processing environment used in a particular department. Density controls are available to increase or decrease exposure. The AEC has a mechanism to terminate exposure, known as a *backup timer*. Once a preselected exposure has been reached, a warning mechanism alerts the technologist that the exposure has been terminated. On newer equipment, the AEC anticipates the required exposure for a given breast. If the exposure necessary to penetrate a patient exceeds the preset exposure limits, the machine will terminate the exposure within the first few milliseconds. This avoids unnecessary exposure to the patient.

Some AECs do not have the ability to "track" patients with extreme differences in glandular (or dense) breast tissue. The AEC should respond to thickness for the same tissue type and the properly selected kVp. The inability of an AEC to react consistently may be due to several factors (2):

1. The characteristics of the screen-film combinations. Some AEC systems may not be able to provide consistent film densities with the limited exposure latitude of modern high-contrast mammography films.
2. The size of the detector. It may be too small to detect the various breast tissue types within the entire breast.
3. The original AECs were not always designed for breast tissue imaging.
4. There may be variable AEC effects due to beam hardening.

Improvements continue to be made to the AECs with the newer mammography units (8). Often, upgrades are available for the "first"-generation AECs.

1. The AECs are better able to compensate for the varying breast tissue types. Design changes have been made to overcome errors caused by the effects of beam hardening.
2. The size of the detector has been increased. The AEC is better able to detect the different breast tissue types.
3. Most of the units have variable detector positions. The detector may be moved after the patient's breast size and/or tissue type are assessed.

4. Some detectors can be electronically controlled. Not only is the detector position selected but a "full AEC" can be selected. The full AEC engages the detector's capacity to cover a larger area.

Equipment has become available whereby the AEC has the ability to compensate for tissue type by altering the target and filtration. Based upon a pre-exposure measurement, after the patient is positioned and compressed, the AEC has an autoselection mechanism that chooses the appropriate anode and filtration.

The AEC has proved to be helpful in those facilities where all of the staff are required to rotate through mammography. In this situation, the image quality can be maintained at some level of consistency. Phototiming has helped to reduce the procedure time. Proper patient positioning is critical when using phototiming. Some patients with abnormal breast parenchyma will require manual exposure. Chapter 6, "Techniques in Screen-Film Mammography," has a further discussion of automatic exposure control.

1.10. Grids

The x-ray beam that exits the breast contains scattered radiation. In order to absorb this, grids are used to improve radiographic image contrast. Grid imaging, in mammography, requires an increase in the exposure by approximately 2.5 times as compared to non-grid exposures (5–7, 9). This will depend on the grid ratio. Improvements in the entire mammography imaging chain promote the increased usage of the grid.

Mammography grids are thinner than the grids used in conventional radiography and have carbon fiber or other low-attenuation interspacing. Two styles of grids are available:

1. Reciprocating bucky or moving grids: The format size can be 18 × 24 cm, 24 × 30 cm, or 24 × 30 cm with an adapter for the 18 × 24 cm cassette. The grid ratio can vary from 3.5:1 to 5:1, with 30 to 50 lines per cm.
2. Stationary grids: These are designed to be placed into some mammography cassettes, grid caps, or a cassette tunnel. They are approximately 1 mm thick and have very fine grid lines. The grid ratio is 3.5:1; 200 lines per inch or 72 lines per centimeter. Stationary grids can obscure fine detail

and are not recommended for high quality modern mammography.

Manufacturers will provide information about the grid ratio and type of grid they use with their equipment.

Although the basic design of the reciprocating bucky has remained similar to those introduced on the first mammography units, improvements continue to be made, such as:

- design improvements in the electronic and mechanical mechanism to reduce grid lines
- "corner molding," which has been added to the outer edges for patient comfort

Reciprocating or moving grids are routinely used for almost all modern high-quality mammography except for magnification views.

The newer technology of the mammography imaging chain allows acceptable exposure levels with the grid.

1.11. Beam-Limiting Devices

Most mammography units today have some type of beam-limiting device available, such as an aperture, diaphragm, cones, or a collimator. The design of the collimator will regulate the size and shape of the x-ray beam. Beam restriction, or collimation, improves the beam quality by helping to eliminate scatter radiation. As the size of the x-ray field decreases, an increase in exposure may be required to maintain a constant image density.

Collimation in mammography is different from that in conventional radiography. In general radiography, all four sides of the film are collimated to irradiate only the region of interest. In mammography, collimation should only be to the size of the image receptor, with care that the field extends just slightly (2% of SID) beyond the image receptor at the chest wall to prevent exclusion of any breast tissue (see Chapter 8, Section 6.5).

The entire film should be exposed (black background). The presence of extraneous light compromises perception of the fine detail. Exposing the entire field does not increase patient dose or significantly increase scatter. Many of the view boxes available incorporate masking devices. Some radiologists prefer to evaluate images with a tunnel or hand-held viewer. Collimation to a small, localized area, as in spot views, will require an increase in exposure factors to maintain a constant image density. The collimation reduces the scattered radiation, which will reduce the image density (see Chapter 6).

1.12. Compression Devices

The compression device is used to apply compression to the patient's breast while a mammogram is made. The compression device must be independent of the tube assembly. Various compression devices are supplied with the purchase of a mammography unit. A spot compression device and compression paddles to correspond to the film format should be included. Other compression paddles such as magnification and localization devices are available. Your equipment manufacturer should be consulted.

The design of the compression plate is very important (Figure 4.4) (1, 9, 10).

1. The flat surface should be parallel to the film receptor. Even compression permits uniform exposure of the entire breast.
2. The lip along the chest wall should be 2 to 4 cm in height.
3. The thickness of the compression device should permit taut compression with minimal discomfort to the patient.
4. The lip should have right angles at the chest wall. Some manufacturers vary the angle slightly for patient comfort.

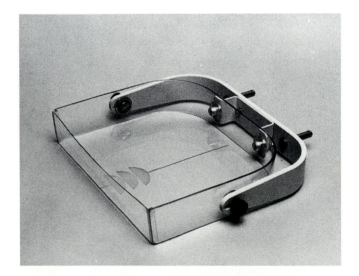

Figure 4.4. Compression device. Reprinted courtesy of LoRad Medical Systems, Danbury, CT.

The design of the lip (both the height and the angle along the chest wall) will make a difference in the final outcome of the imaged examination (1).

1. The lip helps to prevent the posterior and axillary fat from overlapping the body of the breast.
2. The lip affects how the posterior breast tissue is "pulled" into position.
3. The design of the lip helps the actual structural strength of the device itself.

Most units have some type of mechanical compression that can be operated by using a foot pedal with manual backup. A mechanical system frees the technologist and gives him or her an "extra hand" while positioning the patient. The manual backup allows the technologist to complete or perfect the compression after the patient is properly positioned. Some mammography units have a mechanism to set the pressure limits of the mechanical compression. An emergency button is positioned on the unit in case it becomes necessary to release the patient.

A compression scale should be available to monitor the amount of compression administered or provide consistent compression from one breast to the next. The value of compression in screen-film mammography cannot be emphasized enough. This topic is covered in greater detail in Chapter 6.

1.13. Magnification

When the distance between the breast and the image receptor is increased, the area of interest is magnified. Increasing the size of a suspicious lesion on the mammogram may increase the physician's ability to determine a diagnosis altering patient management. The most common magnification factor is 1.5 times. Some units have the ability to perform magnification by 1.6, 1.7, 1.85, or 2 times. The greater the magnification factor, the greater the skin dose to the patient.

To compensate for the reduced resolution resulting from magnification, one must use the smallest focal spot when performing magnification. Failure to select the small focal spot will result in a blurred image. The small focal spot will have a lower mA output, resulting in longer exposure times and thus increasing the chance of patient motion.

Magnification studies reduce scatter. The breast is the source of scattered radiation. Positioning the breast at a point away from the film or increasing the space between the breast and the film takes advantage of the inverse-square law. The intensity of the scattered radiation is reduced because the distance between the film and the object increased. Because of this phenomenon, the grid is unnecessary and should not be used for magnification studies.

Magnification is not recommended for routine imaging. Magnification may be beneficial when (1, 4, 9, 11, 12):

- radiographing the dense or the extremely small breast
- magnifying the surgical site of a patient who has had a lumpectomy
- enlarging the specimen to help the pathologist further evaluate a suspicious lesion or localize an area in question
- evaluating a lesion containing microcalcifications
- further assessing the borders of a lesion
- enlarging an area of interest to increase signal to noise ratio and thus improve the radiologist's ability to perceive detail

Sometimes magnification is used incorrectly. Spot compression views without magnification may be more beneficial to evaluate an area of suspicion. Correctly deciding whether to magnify an area or to use spot compression comes with experience and comfort in performing the procedure.

2. Image Recording

Today a variety of screen-film systems are available for dedicated mammography. Xerography or xero-mammography, popular in the 1970s and 1980s, is declining. New technologies are continuously being discussed and pursued. For example, digital mammography is still being developed in an attempt to achieve the high resolution required in breast imaging. The screen-film systems presently used provide image quality comparable to that of direct-exposure industrial-type film. The dramatic increase in speed has permitted:

- use of a lower kVp which results in higher subject contrast
- a decrease in exposure time, which has resulted in less patient motion and less exposure to the patient
- use of dedicated mammography equipment with improved and smaller focal spot sizes

In this section, the factors contributing to the image recording process are discussed. Those factors include the cassette, the screen-film combination, processing parameters, and darkroom conditions.

2.1. Film Holder

The film holder or cassette (Figure 4.5A and B) is a hard shell protective casing that holds and stores the film during exposure. Various features unique to breast imaging require the film holder or cassette to be designed only for mammography. The cassette must be thin, lightweight, and have excellent screen-film contact. The film holders or cassettes currently designed for mammography should have the following features (13).

1. When the film is placed into the cassette, the position of the film must be as close to the breast surface as possible.
2. The design of the cassette must ensure that the film will be "pulled" close to the chest wall.
3. The cassette must be easy to open.
4. The cassette must be durable.
5. The cassette should have low absorption characteristics to maintain low patient exposures and ensure accurate phototimer response.

Today, two styles of mammography cassettes are available:

1. A black plastic box-holder. The screen is mounted onto a foam layer. When film is placed into this cassette, the film must be positioned manually so it is placed toward the chest wall.
2. A thinner cassette, designed for daylight handling systems, has become available in recent years. This style of cassette automatically positions the film closer to the chest wall and has incorporated an identification system permitting patient information to be photographed onto the film.

The film, screen, and cassette must be aligned correctly in relation to the x-ray beam. Incorrect positioning of the film, screen, or cassette will degrade the image. Patient exposure will increase as a result of repeat exposures taken when the film is improperly loaded upside down into the cassette or the cassette is improperly loaded into the film holder (Figure 4.6).

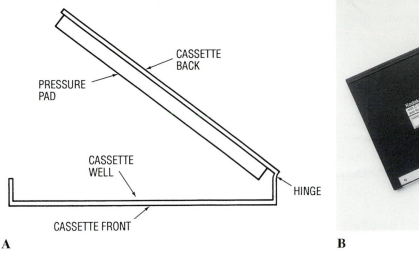

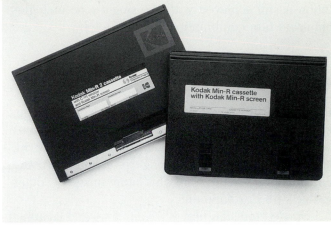

A   **B**

Figure 4.5.   **A.** Cassette line drawing. Reproduced by permission of MTP Press Limited, Lancaster, England, from Jenkins D: Radiographic Photography and Imaging Processes. Copyright® 1980, MTP Press. **B.** Kodak Min-R 2 Cassette and Kodak Min-R Cassette, the two styles of mammography cassette available today. Courtesy of Eastman Kodak Company, Rochester, NY.

2.2. Screens

A screen looks like a piece of white plastic. It is a thin phosphor layer coated onto a support base. Most recent mammography screens are based on the same phosphor, gadolinium oxysulfide, which emits green light when exposed to an x-ray beam. Other improved phosphors—which emit green, blue, or UV light—are being explored for further improvements in image quality.

An intensifying screen is a device that converts the x-ray beam into light: the phosphor absorbs the x-rays and converts the energy to visible or ultraviolet light. The transformation from x-rays to light re-

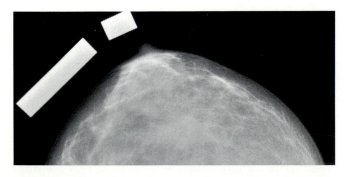

Figure 4.6.   Film placed into the mammography cassette improperly, resulting in an image that appears underexposed.

duces patient exposures because the film is much more sensitive to light than to x-rays. A single screen is used as a back screen, with the film placed in intimate contact and on top of the screen. This configuration takes advantage of the highest emission and lowest scatter from the screen.

Introduction of higher-speed screens reduce patient exposure approximately 40% over the standard screens. This increase in speed not only permits a lower dose for magnification studies and grid work but is helpful to reduce exposure for those patients whose breasts are difficult to penetrate. Although these higher-speed screens result in some compromise in image quality, many radiologists find the image quality of the faster screens acceptable for use in screening and routine mammography. These faster screens combined with a high-speed single-emulsion film provide approximately the same dose reduction as a double-screen system (14).

A double-screen film system was introduced in 1986. In view of the later developments of the faster single screen, the only advantages of a double-screen film system are as follows (1, 14):

- the film is less susceptible to imaging dust and dirt
- the double-emulsion films do not require extended processing times to develop optimum contrast and speed

Several studies have documented that the best resolution is still achieved with the single-screen single-emulsion film combination.

2.3. Film

Film is used to record the image, display the image, and provide archival storage. Once the interactions occur between the x-ray beam, the patient, the grid, and the screen, a latent image is formed into the emulsion layer of the film. This latent image becomes visible with development.

Single-emulsion film is made of several layers:

1. The film base is a transparent plastic material.
2. On both sides of the film base are gelatin layers that are necessary for the adhesion of the various other layers of the film.
3. The emulsion layer is only coated on one side of the film base.
4. The emulsion layer contains silver halide crystals that are inherently sensitive to ultraviolet and blue light.
5. If the film is to be used with a green-emitting screen, then the silver halide grains must be sensitized with a green-absorbing dye. In this layer, also, a variety of chemical compounds are included that ensure stability, low fog, and fast processing.
6. The emulsion layer is protected by a top coating that is an antiabrasive layer.
7. On the back side of the film, the dark side, opposite the emulsion side of the film, an antihalation layer helps to prevent light scatter and improves resolution. This layer also prevents the film from curling during processing.

Special care must be taken to ensure that the emulsion side of the film is in contact with the screen (see Figure 4.6). Manufacturers notch their film so correct placement of the film can be accomplished by feel in the darkroom. Some cassette manufacturers have included a marker in the cassette so technologists can align the notch of the film with the marker. Some cassettes have a button indicating whether or not the film is loaded in the cassette. The screen and film are housed in a dedicated mammography cassette (see Section 2.1).

Selection of the appropriate screen-film system is based on personal preference. At no time must the image quality or the patient dose be compromised. Most importantly, the screen-film system of choice

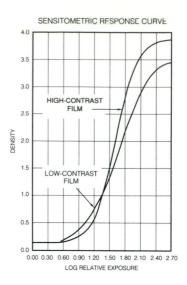

Figure 4.7. Characteristic curve demonstrating a mammography film high in contrast versus a film low in contrast.

must be designed for mammography and should preferably be a single-screen film system (9).

For mammography, a film high in contrast is preferred. Film characteristics, such as speed and contrast are described by the characteristic curve (also called the H&D curve). It shows the relationship between the exposure a film has received and the corresponding optical density after processing. The optical density is a measure of the blackening of the film. The characteristic curve describes the film for the particular processing environment it was developed in, including the processor, chemistry, time, and temperature. The characteristic curve does not depend upon the x-ray beam quality or the screens as long as the same phosphor emission spectrum is used. This means that the shape of the curve does not change with exposure factors such as kVp and mAs; these factors only change the position of the curve along the exposure axis (horizontal).

The characteristic curve may be plotted to compare two different film types, to compare the same film processed in different conditions, or to monitor the daily processing conditions. The film with the steepest slope in the straight-line portion of the curve has the highest "overall" contrast (Figure 4.7). The toe is the region of the lightest areas or "whites" on the film, corresponding with "high-density" breast tissue. The shoulder represents the darkest areas on the film or the "low-density" breast tissue. Toe and shoulder contrast also influence the overall contrast of the image (see Figure 4.8).

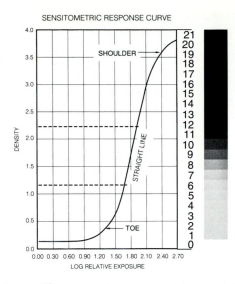

Figure 4.8. Characteristic curve pointing out the toe, straight line, and shoulder portion of the curve.

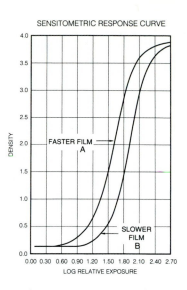

Figure 4.9. Characteristic curve showing two films of different system speeds.

Film contrast, as described above, should never be considered as the only factor determining the image system contrast. The image system contrast, as perceived on the view box or on the mammogram, comprises all the factors contributing to the final image (see Chapter 6, Section 2.1), including viewing conditions.

In Figure 4.9, the film in A will be faster than the film in B; that is, less exposure is required to produce the same density.

When comparing two films having the same speed and the same inherent sharpness and exposed with the same screen, generally the film with the higher contrast will be perceived as demonstrating more detail. High-contrast films, however, have limited exposure latitude (see Chapter 6, "Techniques in Screen-Film Mammography").

2.4. Processing Conditions

The film must pass many steps before the final image is obtained. Once a latent image is formed, the film must be processed. Improper processing is the most common pitfall in mammography. Today, processing is usually done by an automatic processor. The processing conditions affect both the position and the shape of the characteristic curve—that is, the speed and the contrast.

Dedicated processing is strongly encouraged (Figure 4.10). It is not uncommon to find a department sharing a processor using several other kinds of

film. An alternative to this problem may be to have all single-emulsion films developed in a separate processor. This processor must have the parameters optimized for mammography, keeping in mind the screen-film combination used and the film manufacturer's recommendations. Optimizing the processing conditions is difficult, considering the complexity of the processor. Film must pass through many steps before the final image is obtained.

1. The film first travels through the developer section of the processor. When the exposed film is placed into the developer solution, a visible image is produced.
2. Next the film travels through the fixer section of the processor. In the fixer section, development is stopped, and the image is made permanent by removing the unexposed and the undeveloped silver halide from the film.
3. The film then travels to the wash section. The wash is designed to remove the chemicals remaining in the layers after processing.
4. Finally, the film travels through the dryer section. Here the film is dried and prepared for viewing.

During processing, within both the developer and the fixer section, a variety of chemical reactions take place. As a result of this, the original solutions are depleted. To maintain the level of original activity and not sacrifice the image quality, one must periodically replenish the solutions.

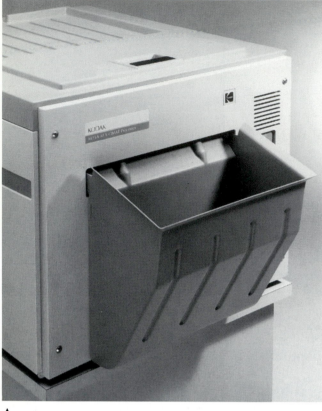

A

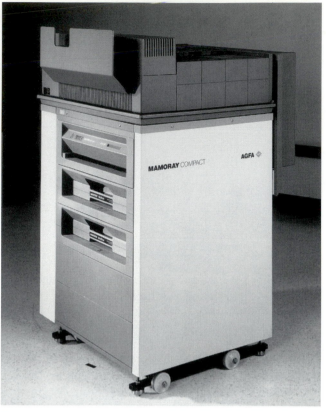

B

Figure 4.10. Dedicated processing is strongly encouraged. Processing parameters must be optimized to the film manufacturer's guidelines. Facilities may choose either of the following:
A. A smaller processor designed for mammography such as Kodak M35A-M X-OMAT Processor. Courtesy of Eastman Kodak Company, Rochester, NY.

B. A daylight film-handling system such as the Mamoray Compact, which may be placed in the mammography room because a darkroom is not required. Courtesy of Agfa Division, Bayer Corporation, Ridgefield Park, NJ.

Contrast, speed, and thus the perceptible detail can be modified or affected by the following processing conditions (2, 4, 15):

1. developer temperature
2. developer time
3. processor maintenance:
   - chemical activity
   - agitation
   - cleanliness

The developer temperature is the temperature of the solutions in the processor, especially the developer solutions. Most mammography films must be processed in developer solutions that remain constant at 35°C (95°F) (2, 4, 15).

1. A decrease in the developer temperature below that recommended may result in:

- an increase in exposure to obtain the desired image density
- a decrease in image contrast
- an increase in the radiation dose to the patient
- increased wear of the x-ray tube

2. If the developer temperature is increased above that recommended:
   - the film speed may increase
   - the film fog and quantum mottle may increase, thus increasing the radiographic noise
   - the stability of the developer may also be affected

The developer time is the length of time the film is in the developer. In the standard 90-s processor, the film is usually in the developer for 20 to 25 s. The development time, sometimes called the immersion time, can be extended to further improve the speed and contrast. The developer temperature should remain at 35°C (95°F) when the developer time is extended. The effects of extended or "pushed" processing will vary with the film manufacturer's recommendations for a particular film (Figure 4.11) (8, 13, 15–17).

Increasing the developer time can be done either by slowing down the entire processor or by gearing down the developer section (16). With certain emulsion types, the advantages to extending the developer time are:

- increase in film speed, which lowers patient dose and reduces patient motion
- shorter exposure times, which equate with longer tube life
- increase in film contrast (15)

Disadvantages of extended processing include the risk of increasing the film fog and increased processor artifacts. At all times it is best to optimize the

processing environment to obtain the optimum contrast and speed from the film.

Processing is also influenced by the type of developer, the agitation, and replenishment of the chemical solutions. During development, a thin layer of chemicals stagnates on the surface of the film. During this stage the chemical solution progresses from fresh to exhausted. The old processing solutions become too weak and underdevelop the films. Thus, it is important to have the replenishment rates set to maintain the desired chemical activity. The exact amount of replenishment depends on the number and the size of the films processed as well as the developer temperature. Automatic processors have a monitoring system to replenish solutions as needed. Confer with the film-chemistry-processor manufacturer(s) to determine the correct replenishment rates. Problems in maintaining stable sensitometry will occur especially in low-volume facilities; whereby insufficient quantities of film are processed through the processor and minimize oxidation.

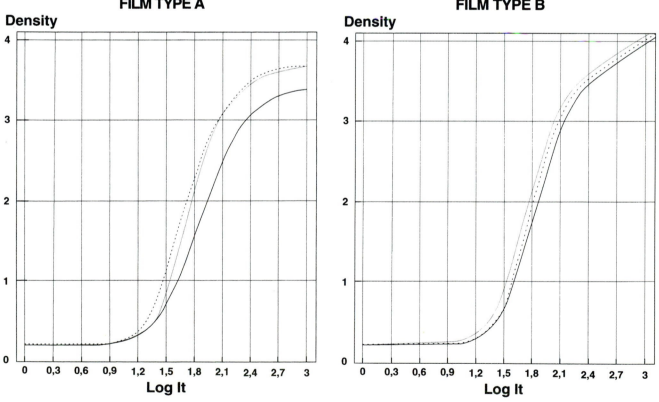

Figure 4.11. Processing dynamics of two different mammography film types. The characteristic curves demonstrate that film A responds to variations in the processing system: chemistry, developer time, developer temperature, or replenishment rates more quickly than seen with film type B.

Solutions must be replaced according to the manufacturer's recommendations. Authors have stated that solutions must be replaced every 1 to 2 weeks (15,16). When a new chemical solution is poured on top of the old, the chemicals become more diluted or oxidized. A small amount of oxidized chemicals acts like a catalyst and oxidizes the fresh chemicals more quickly. If film usage and replenishment rates are sufficiently high to completely replace the solutions in the developer and fixer tanks in 1 or 2 days, then dumping and replacing chemicals may be unnecessary over long periods of time, so that the sensitometric variations usually associated with startup conditions can be minimized.

An area not usually discussed with regard to processing and chemistry for mammography application is the water. If a particular geographic area has a lot of dirt or minerals in the water, the debris will work its way into the system. The debris will get mixed into the chemical solutions, travel to the processor, and lodge itself onto the rollers or in the chemical tanks. This may potentially cause artifacts that may look like microcalcifications.

> **Suggestion:** When installing a processor for mammography, add a water filter to the water line into the department as well as filters out of the chemical mixers. These filters should be cleaned monthly or as required by high sediment content in the water.

Some geographic areas may experience problems with a buildup of algae in water tanks. In such conditions it may be necessary to add algicides or filters to reduce the potential for organic growth in the wash tanks.

Too often, processor maintenance is overlooked. A processor is like a car. Those processors used for developing mammography film should be treated like an expensive sports car. Daily monitoring of the processor is the best method to determine if any changes have occurred. Daily processor maintenance should include:

- sensitometry to include film speed (mid-density), film contrast (density difference), and base plus fog
- monitoring of developer temperature
- cleaning of crossover rollers (*Note:* ask your processor service company to indicate which rollers should be cleaned and to demonstrate how the roller should be rinsed off each day.)

The processor should be thoroughly evaluated at least once a month. In those facilities where few patients are examined, it is especially important to keep a watchful eye on the processor environment.

Improper and inadequate developing is a common problem in mammography. Adjunctive methods, such as use of a lower kVp or switching to a higher-contrast film, are sometimes used to improve poor contrast but without resolving the real problem—improper processing.

2.5. System Speed and Reciprocity Law Failure

System speed directly affects patient dose. Improvements in screen-film technology and the dedicated mammography exposure unit have helped to reduce patient exposure. These advances help the technologist to properly penetrate the more glandular tissue type breast. One must take care to ensure that the exposure to the low-attenuation breast is not too short.

System speed can be maximized by combining a high-speed film with fast screens. The drawback of high-speed screen-film systems is the question of the acceptable noise levels and sharpness on the final image. It is important to pair both the film and the screen to provide an acceptable system speed without compromising image quality. As a rule, the system speed is optimized when the film is processed according to the recommendations of the manufacturers.

Recent improvements in x-ray tube technology have also permitted reduction in patient exposure. Higher mA output and improved generators (high-voltage wave form) have increased the quality of radiation.

The influence of reciprocity failure is often overlooked. The reciprocity law (3, 8, 18) states that the film speed varies with exposure time. Ideally, two identical mAs exposures should provide the same optical density on a film. When reciprocity failure occurs, additional exposure becomes necessary to provide the desired density on the film. Exposures ranging from 0.1 to 2 s may result in a 20 to 30% speed difference. For example,

Example #1: 28 kVp, 200 mA, 0.25 s
Example #2: 28 kVp, 20 mA, 2.5 s

although both exposures result in 50 mAs. Example #2 might require increasing the exposure by approximately 30% to obtain the same optical density as Example #1. If the increase in exposure is necessary, the exposure time will be increased from 2.5 s to 3.25 s or approximately 70 mAs. The exposure time is seldom under operator control. The technologist must try to keep patient exposure as low as possible. When necessary, take advantage of a higher kVp, alter the target and/or filtration material, or use a faster screen-film combination. Most modern AEC systems provide automatic correction for film reciprocity failure.

2.6. Darkroom

The sensitivity of single-emulsion film demands proper film handling and darkroom maintenance. The darkroom must be used for its specific purpose and kept spotless. The darkroom should not become the department storage closet. The bench tops, processor feed trays, and any other equipment must be kept free of dust, dried chemicals, or other debris. At no time should anyone smoke or eat in the darkroom. Cleanliness cannot be overemphasized.

> **Suggestion:** Wet-mop the floor daily. Wipe down the countertops with antistatic solution.

The darkroom must be properly ventilated. Proper room temperature (from 50 to 70°F) and humidity (from 40 to 65%) must be maintained. The air supply should be sufficient to remove any chemical fumes. The processing environment must be maintained. Care must be taken to clean up chemical spills and splashes.

The correct safelight filter and the correct light bulb and wattage must be placed in the darkroom. The spectral sensitivity of the film must be taken into account when selecting safelight filters (18).

> **Suggestion:** The most common safelight is the Kodak GBX-2. The bulb is usually 7 1/2 to 15 W.

The safelight should be positioned at least 4 ft away from the work area or the feed tray. A safelight test should be performed when replacing the bulb or the filter.

Care must be taken to ensure that the light leaks around the doors, pass boxes, and processors are eliminated. Light leaks will result in a loss of contrast on the final image. In mammography especially, this can destroy a quality examination. Chapter 8, Section 10.1, describes how to determine if this is a problem.

The film must be stored correctly. Film should be kept in a light-tight container such as a film bin. Small departments may prefer to use the small plastic film boxes that are commercially available. It is not considered good practice to keep an open box of film on the countertop.

2.7. Film Fog

Film fog will degrade the image quality. Uniform film fog leaves an unwanted density on the film and may be caused by chemical contamination, poor storage conditions, or external exposure from a safelight or unwanted x-ray. Chemical fog due to contaminated chemicals can also deteriorate the image.

Film fog can best be demonstrated on the characteristic curve (see Figure 4.12).

1. The "whites" on the image are degraded by a higher fog in the toe region of the curve.
2. The "blacks" are imaged lower in contrast.
3. There is an apparent gain in speed.

Any alterations that influence the characteristic curve and minimize the high-contrast appearance will result in suboptimal image quality.

Too often, the film and processing environment are taken for granted. Care must be taken to maintain stability in this area to provide consistent image recording.

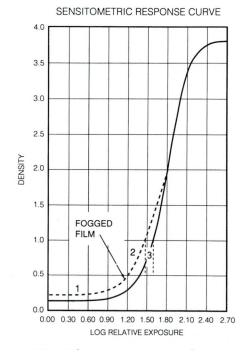

Figure 4.12. Characteristic curve demonstrating the effects of fog on the film.

3. Image Quality

Every woman who has a mammogram deserves to have an examination that provides high image quality. Such terms as *detailed, sharp, crisp, brilliant*, and *pretty* are used to convey the idea of quality. What constitutes a quality mammogram?

The radiologist's opinion of image quality is based upon personal preference, experience, and knowledge of the procedure. This opinion is subjective. The requirements to visualize a microcalcification in a fatty breast as opposed to a very glandular, dense breast are different. Image quality determines the accuracy with which the various structures are recorded and the abnormalities detected. It becomes necessary to define various components of the imaging chain and how these properties affect the final mammogram. Some technical factors intrinsic to image quality are the inherent properties of the mammographic equipment and the screen-film systems, as discussed in Sections 1 and 2. Other factors, however, are controlled by the technologist.

In this section, technical factors influencing image quality and their interactions to produce a diagnostic image will be discussed. Mammographic image quality can be divided into two major components (Figure 4.13): radiographic sharpness and radiographic noise.

3.1. Radiographic Sharpness

Sharpness is the ability to identify or image the edges of objects such as microcalcifications. The perceived sharpness in a mammogram is the function of *radiographic contrast* and *radiographic blurring.*

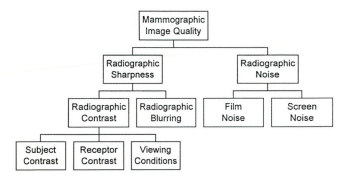

Figure 4.13. Components of mammographic image quality.

3.1.1. Radiographic Contrast

Radiographic contrast is the density difference within the various breast architectures (parenchyma) and is the product of subject contrast and receptor contrast.

Subject contrast is the variation of intensity of the x-ray beam leaving the breast. Each patient's breast has different tissue types and thickness, resulting in a large range of subject contrast. Factors influencing subject contrast that can be controlled by the operator are as follows:

1. The appropriate kVp setting should be chosen. The selected kVp setting should be low enough to provide the highest contrast but high enough to properly penetrate the breast.
2. The scatter radiation should be reduced by proper collimation. The breast should be vigorously compressed and the grid should be used (see Section 1).

Factors that the technologist often does not have any control over but that do influence subject contrast are the patient (tissue type, density, and thickness) and the equipment selected (the target material, filters, and exit window).

Receptor contrast is the inherent contrast coming from the design of the screen and film system selected. The screen-film combination is usually predetermined. By optimizing the processing conditions as directed by the manufacturer, one will optimize receptor contrast. In mammography, the processing environment can be the weak link of an imaging system if it is not optimized to the manufacturer's recommendations (See Section 2 in this chapter and Chapter 9, Section 8).

Receptor contrast can be too low or too high and will appear as under- or overexposure. The AEC exposures must be optimized to the screen, film, cassette, and processing conditions employed at a given facility. Uniform fog, as a result of improper storage, improper safelights, and light leaks, is often difficult to trace and is very degrading to the receptor contrast. The technologist can make sure the receptor contrast is optimized by:

- performing daily quality-control on the processor (Chapter 9, Section 8.5)
- making sure the AEC is correctly calibrated
- storing the film as recommended by the manufacturer

Radiographic viewing conditions strongly affect the viewer's ability to detect density differences on a film. Because of the expanded range of film densities (expanded dynamic range) available with modern mammography films, careful attention to viewing conditions is essential for high quality mammography. Use of appropriate viewing conditions is one of the most frequently neglected elements essential for high-density mammography.

3.1.2. Radiographic Blurring

An image with sharpness, or definition, will provide the radiologist with the desired detail. If a mammogram is not sharp, the patient might not get a proper diagnosis. Factors that influence radiographic blurring are motion blur, geometric blur, and receptor blur. Some of these factors can be controlled by the operator.

Motion blur, whether voluntary or involuntary, can be controlled with proper compression and the lowest possible exposure time. The technologist must apply vigorous compression. As discussed in Chapter 6, Section 1, compression not only immobilizes the breast and spreads the breast tissue laterally but also enhances subject contrast. Maximum compression reduces the breast thickness, and thus the x-ray beam has less distance to travel to reach the film, reducing scatter radiation. When breast thickness is reduced, exposure times are reduced.

Geometric blur is equipment-related. The technologist cannot control the physics of the equipment. During the purchasing process of a dedicated mammography machine, the geometry of the equipment selected must be optimized for breast imaging. The factors that will influence geometric blur are the focal spot size (Section 1.3), the SID (Section 1.4), and the object-to-film distance (Section 1.5). When the focal spot size is influenced by the mA selection, the technologist should always use the smallest focal spot size possible for the procedure being performed (see Chapter 6, Section 2.2.4).

Receptor blur is dependent on the intensifying screen selected. Films today have inherently higher resolution than that of the intensifying screens, so the differences in resolution seen among screen-film systems come predominantly from the different screens used.

The technologists do not have control over the various physical properties of the screen-film system used in their departments. These factors, such as the

phosphor thickness coated onto the screen, are inherent within the design of the receptor. The technologist can, however, monitor the screen-film contact. As cassettes and screens age, the contact may begin to deteriorate. If poor screen-film contact is suspected, a screen-film contact mesh wire exposure should be taken. Poor screen-film contact may result as a blurred area on the radiograph (Chapter 9, Section 7.4).

3.2. Radiographic Noise

Radiographic noise, always present in an image, can easily be seen as the density variation that occurs on a uniformly exposed and developed film. A distinction must be made between the *radiographic mottle* and the noise due to *artifacts.*

3.2.1. Radiographic Mottle

Radiographic mottle in practical applications has two major components: film graininess and quantum mottle. With the increased film speeds introduced in the last decade, film graininess is gaining importance in the total noise. Additional film speed generally comes from the larger silver halide emulsion crystals used in the emulsion. Unfortunately, increased film speed, whether coming from film design or such parameters as extended processing, reduces the number of absorbed x-ray quanta (photons) required to achieve a given film optical density. The use of fewer x-ray photons to make the image increases quantum mottle.

Note: There are two significant artifacts in mammography that may be diagnosed as radiographic mottle not discussed above. They are processor roller mottle or filtration (x-ray target) nonuniformity. Mottle imparted to the film image by uneven pressure from dirty or damaged rollers is frequently a significant source for image noise. Mottle imparted to the film image by nonuniformity of the filter within the x-ray equipment tube may be mistaken for processor mottle. Care must be taken to determine the source of the mottle.

3.2.2. Artifacts

Artifacts hinder the quality of the final image. There are a great variety of artifacts coming from film handling, exposure fog, or processing. Three categories of artifacts are discussed:

1. Screen artifacts
2. Film artifacts
3. System artifacts

Screen artifacts are among the most significant problems in mammography.

1. Objects will cast a shadow onto the final image. For example,
   - dust
   - dirt
   - hair
   - other small foreign bodies within the cassette
2. Abrasions are a result of the loading and unloading of the film.
3. Excessive cleaning of the screen surface will cause screen wear.

Film artifacts are a result of poor maintenance or handling. As long as the operator handles the film properly in and outside of the darkroom and the processor is well maintained, the artifacts can be minimized. Other problems causing film artifacts are as follows:

1. Film fog will deteriorate image quality.
2. Film handling artifacts deteriorate image quality. Examples of film handling artifacts are:
   - pressure artifacts—dark crescent marks on the finish film
   - static electricity—humidity and proper ventilation should be maintained in the darkroom
   - foreign chemicals—fingerprints, for example
   (Individuals who have perspiration problems should wear white cotton gloves while handling film.)
3. Improper processing and malfunctioning of the automatic processors can be detrimental in mammography. Very small randomized artifacts, generally generated in the processing rollers, are often overlooked and thought to be the film noise or quantum mottle (see Chapter 10, Section 2). A few of the problems that will occur are:
   - streaks, mottle, and "chewed up" films
   - processing solutions not mixed well
   - dirty rollers

In mammography, *system artifacts* will degrade image quality, which may delay the proper diagnosis for the patient. Some of the artifacts seen stem from

- insufficient cleanliness of the mammography equipment
- patient anatomy superimposed on the radiograph
- flaws in the compression device, grid, or image receptor

Note: Any imperfections or irregularity in a moving grid will introduce noise patterns that are frequently a significant cause of image noise in mammography.

4. Summary

Image quality is determined by the total effect of the imaging chain on the final appearance on the radiograph. Some of the factors that contribute to the final image are determined by the intrinsic parameters of the imaging chain. Factors such as selecting the correct kVp for the patient and correctly applying compression are controlled by the operator.

To provide the patient with the best possible mammogram requires three key factors: (1) dedicated mammography equipment, (2) screen-film combination with dedicated processing, and (3) well-trained personnel. Two of these components are discussed in this chapter.

1. It is imperative to perform mammography with a dedicated mammography x-ray machine in which the physics and design are exclusive for breast imaging.
2. The screen-film combination must be designed for mammography. The weak link in mammography is still the processing. To optimize image quality, manufacturers' guidelines for their screen-film combination should be followed.

Acknowledgement: I would like to thank Lee Kitt, Ph.D., for his assistance and valuable input in this chapter.

References

1. Harrill C, White S, Gillespie K, et al. Evaluation of dual-screen, dual emulsion mammography system. AJR 1989;152:483–486.

2. Helvie MA, Heang-Ping C: Breast thickness in routine mammograms—Effect on image quality and radiation dose. AJR 1994;163:1371–1374.

3. Curry TS, Dowdey JE, Murry RC. Christensen's Physics of Diagnostic Radiology, 4th ed. Philadelphia: Lea & Febiger; 1990:4:137–148.

4. Jenkins D. Radiographic Photography and Imaging Processes. Baltimore: University Park Press; 1980:36–47, 59–89, 127–149, 166–189, 222–236.

5. Haus AG. Screen-Film Mammography Update: X-Ray Units, Breast Compression Grids, Screen-Film Characteristics and Radiation Dose. Rochester, NY: Eastman Kodak; 1984.

6. Haus AG. Screen Film Mammography Update. Rochester, NY: Eastman Kodak; 1986.

7. Haus AG. Recent advances in screen-film mammography. Radiol Clin North Am 1987;25:913–928.

8. Haus AG. Technologic improvements in screen-film mammography. Radiology 1990;174:628–637.

9. Kimme-Smith C, Bassett LW, Gold RH: Film screen mammography X-ray tube anodes: Molybdenum vs tungsten. Med Phys 1989;16:279–283.

10. Logan WW. Screen-Film Mammography. New York: Grune & Stratton; 1979;61-72.

11. National Council on Radiation Protection and Measurements. Mammography: A User's Guide. Bethesda, MD: NCRP 1986(NCRP no. 85):14–27, 57–70.

12. Sickles EA. Further experience with microfocal spot magnification in mammography in the assessment of clustered breast microcalcifications. Radiology 1980;137:9–14.

13. Eklund GW, Surratt D. Extended developer processing time. Admin Radiol 1989;April:22–23.

14. Bassett L, Kimme-Smith C, Gold R, et al. New mammography screen film combinations: Imaging characteristics and radiation dose. AJR 1990;154:713–719.

15. Bassett LW, Gold RH, Kimme-Smith C, Moier C, Rothschild PA. Mammographic film—Processor temperature, development time, and chemistry: Effect on dose, contrast, and noise. AJR 1989;152:35–40.

16. Dean PB, Tabar L. Quality aspects on mammography. Medicamundi 1984;29:71–75.

17. Haus AG, Tabar L. Processing of mammographic films: Technical and clinical consideration. Radiology 1989;173:65–69.

18. Health Sciences Markets Division. The Fundamentals of Radiology, 12th ed. Rochester, NY: Eastman Kodak; 1980:14–106.

19. Sickles EA. Dedicated Mammography Equipment. Categorical course on Mammography. Presented at ACR in Los Angeles; 1984:1–6.

20. American College of Radiology Committee on Quality Assurance in Mammography. Mammography: Mammography Quality Control. Reston, VA: American College of Radiology, 1994.

21. Sickles EA, Weber WN. High-contrast mammography with a moving grid: Assessment of clinical utility. AJR 1986;146:1137–1139.

22. Thunberg SJ. The effect of different anode/filter combinations on image quality and glandular dose. Prepublication manuscript. August 1994.

23. Zamenhof RG, Homer MJ. Equipment mammography: Physical principles. Appl Radiol 1984; September/October:86–99.

5

What Mammography Means to the Patient and the Technologist

Mammography has been an important media topic since the early 1980s. Statistics are continually cited; for example, we are informed that the incidence of breast cancer is on the rise. Until the coming of the American College of Radiology (ACR) and the Mammography Quality Standards Act (MQSA), the attitude toward mammography among most radiologists and administrators was one of avoidance. The least-skilled technologist was assigned to the mammography room; the newest radiologist was assigned the unpleasant task of reading the films; administrators resisted mammography and were unsure how to treat the "charging elephant." The medical community still cannot agree on guidelines for screening mammography.

At one time, only a handful of equipment manufacturers made dedicated mammography machines. Now there are over thirty different pieces of equipment on the market. The MQSA has defined the educational and performance criteria for the breast imaging team. Radiologists coming out of residency are required, as of 1990, to take boards that include mammography. The value of dedicated technologists has been recognized. Finally, administration has realized that mammography is not going away; it is here to stay and is *growing!*

Not only the medical community but also lay people are taking mammography seriously. Women are becoming more educated about the procedure, and they have higher expectations. In this chapter, the psychology of mammography and its effects on both the patient and the technologist are discussed.

Screening and diagnostic procedures and the impact upon the patient are reviewed. Also, the role of the technologist is established.

1. Psychology of Mammography

Psychology is defined by Webster as the science of behavior, or the study of interactions between humans and the social environment. In mammography, the interaction occurs between the patient, the technologist, the referring physician, the radiologist, and potentially the surgeon and the oncologist. This does not include, of course, the interaction among friends, family, the media, and the general public. Interaction can be positive or negative.

Many publications discuss the differences between screening mammography and diagnostic mammography. It does not matter which approach to breast disease a facility selects; the image quality in both scenarios must be maintained at the same high image-quality standards. The biggest difference between a screening facility and a diagnostic facility is how the patients will be evaluated. In a true screening facility, the patient volume is high, as the patients are radiographed to segregate those who may have potential problems. If it is determined that a patient requires further evaluation, he or she is directed to a diagnostic facility or scheduled to have a diagnostic workup.

How does this affect the patient and the technologist? Too often, demands are placed upon a facility to increase patient throughput. Patients may be scheduled every 10 to 15 min. Even with this type of scheduling the technologist is required to have the radiologist review the films and take additional views, perform a needle localization in the middle of a busy schedule, or take specimen films for the operating room. These extra demands place undue stress or additional burden on the technologist and the patient. The entire atmosphere and attitudes of all involved become very hurried.

A facility that performs mammography must define the type of services it will provide to the community and then develop the protocol for handling the patients. A *screening* mammogram is an examination used to detect unsuspected breast cancer at an early stage in asymptomatic women. The patient receives a two-view-per-breast mammogram and is then dismissed. The technologist may check the film for radiographic quality; however, it is not uncommon for the screening mammographic images to be batch processed at a later point. If the results of the examination are suspicious, additional films may be required. The patient is called back to a diagnostic facility or to the original facility on a day when diagnostic procedures are performed. A *diagnostic* mammogram (sometimes known as problem-solving or consultative mammogram) is an examination to follow up on those patients who have been sighted or diagnosed with potential problems. The scheduling of diagnostic patients should are usually performed under the on-site supervision of a qualified physician. The schedule should permit ample time to accommodate multiple views that may be required for the diagnostic examination.

When a physician refers a patient for a mammogram, he or she should communicate with the patient about the type of facility the patient will visit or should give the patient a choice. The entire mammography chain and the procedure are too often a mystery to many patients. When patients, through patient education, know what to expect, they will feel more in control. A patient who is comfortable and feels in control of the situation will be more cooperative and relaxed, thus making the mammogram easier for the technologist to do. Never must image quality suffer because the facility is a screening center and not a diagnostic center.

2. The Patient

Women still do not understand the single greatest weapon available to them in the detection of Breast Cancer. Many patients are apprehensive about mammography and undergoing the procedure. The lack of education and positive communication to prepare a woman for the examination is the major contributor. First, as many women may remember, 20 years ago everyone worried about radiation to the breast. Although much of the radiation scare has been alleviated, people are still concerned. Second, mammography has been exploited by the media. The sensationalism with which the media have treated mammography has misled the patients by not giving them complete and accurate information. The media have focused on the negative and not the positive aspects of this procedure. For example, shortly after the second generation of mammography equipment was introduced, a woman's letter appeared in the "Ann Landers" column criticizing the procedure and complaining of her terrible experience. Unfortunately, bad news travels faster than good news. Third, too many women have truly had a terrible experience during a mammogram. Too often, the woman is rushed through the procedure, much like someone having a chest x-ray taken. Chest x-ray films are usually routine, but in a woman's mind, the

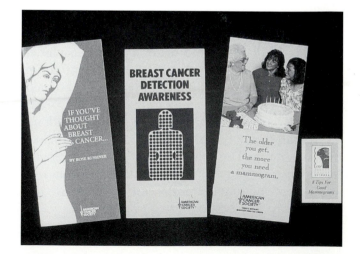

Figure 5.1. A sample of patient education literature that is available for patients to read while waiting for their mammograms or at home. Reprint courtesy of the American Cancer Society, Atlanta, Georgia.

mammogram often suggests that something may be wrong with her. If a woman does have a bad experience, she may not return for a follow-up exam the next year. That is a potential injustice to the quality of the woman's life.

Mammography must be a positive experience. Seven in eight women do not get breast cancer. The mammogram must be regarded as a control method to reduce mortality due to breast cancer, and women must learn to treat the procedure as a routine physical exam, such as a Pap (Papanicolaou) smear. Some facilities go to great lengths and expense to develop a nice, relaxing atmosphere for their patients. For example:

1. The waiting room looks like an elaborate living room.
2. The color scheme throughout the department is coordinated to provide a soft, comfortable, quiet, and peaceful environment.
3. The room for patient education includes a monitor and videotapes as well as breast models so that patients can learn to perform breast self-examination (BSE) and develop confidence in their technique.
   - Brochures can be designed to match the decor of the breast center. Such groups as the ACS have patient education pamphlets available.
   - Shower cards are often given to the women to serve as reminders and refresher guides on how to perform BSE.
   - Visual aids such as radiographs showing good versus bad compression can help patients to understand the procedure.
4. Amenities are available for the patient's added comfort.
   - Washcloths and towels with which to wash off deodorant
   - Gowns designed to allow one breast to be bared while covering the remainder of the patient's chest
   - Deodorant and hair spray for the patient once the exam is completed

The media, with the arrival of the MQSA, have begun to "educate" patients regarding their share of the responsibility when obtaining a mammogram. The patient is told to ask her breast imaging facility about its FDA certification, the personnel training, and/or qualifications and about the facility itself. Each patient has her own anxiety, stress, and unrest surrounding the procedure. She may be concerned for her life: "Am I going to die?" Or she may be afraid that she will be disfigured by breast surgery. Fear of the unknown is difficult for all of us.

3. The Technologist

In mammography, the manner in which the technologist conducts herself or himself leaves a lasting impression upon the patient. The first requirement for a mammography technologist is the ability to speak to the patient while being compassionate. At a time when most x-ray departments are short-staffed, the last thing a technologist needs is more to do. A smile, however, takes less energy than a frown. The technologist should greet the patient pleasantly; first impressions are lasting impressions.

Once in the mammography room, the technologist must conduct herself or himself in a positive and polished manner. The technologist should explain the procedure to the patient, especially if this is the patient's first experience. Efforts should be made to describe compression: the value of compression and what the patient may expect during compression. Never should the words hurt or pain be used during the explanation with the patient. The patient should be allowed to feel in control during the procedure.

The technologist should be prepared to counteract any negative impressions the patient may express. To neutralize those impressions, it is important to remember that actions speak louder than words. If the patient has been told one thing by the technologist but is treated differently, the negativity she may feel has not been dissipated. If time permits, the technologist should take this opportunity to educate the patient. Knowledge is a powerful tool.

A technologist's appearance and body language say a lot to the patient. A technologist who conducts herself or himself in a confident, friendly manner will give a positive impression. Patients can sense competence. A reassured patient is easier to work with. The patient should be treated the way one would want one's mother or oneself to be treated.

It is beneficial for a technologist to have the ability to identify the patient's emotional state. The technologist must learn to listen to what the patient is saying. Also, the technologist must know the fine balance between being supportive for the procedure and deciding how to direct the patient when additional support services may be necessary; for example, referring the patient to a hospice group. Every patient's threshold of pain varies. Something as simple as lowering the compression device a little more slowly may be more comforting to the patient.

Consistency and high image quality are best ensured when several well-trained, interested technologists are assigned to mammography. When technologists rotate through the mammography section, quality suffers, not only radiographic quality but the quality of patient care.

The departmental administration must be prepared to prevent the burnout often experienced by the mammography technologists. In departments where many patients are examined, the burnout problem is more likely to occur. A well-trained backup mammography technologist should be part of the department's staff planning. Those technologists who are all alone or need to be self-motivated should keep in mind one major factor: they are making a major contribution to women's health. The radiologist reads the films the technologist provides him or her. *Anyone who saves one life has given someone the gift of life.*

3.1. Role of the Mammography Technologist

The role of the technologist will depend upon the size of the mammography department. If only one mammographer is working in the department, the suggestions below will be her or his responsibility. If several individuals are involved, the ideas mentioned below will help the department run smoothly. A chief technologist should be assigned the responsibility for supervising the mammography section.

1. The supervisor should assume the role of monitoring the quality assurance program.
2. She or he should supervise other technologists doing the mammography procedures.
3. The supervisor should supervise and assume quality control for the images being produced in the department. Any dissatisfaction with image quality must be communicated to the technologists.
4. The supervisor must be available to make suggestions or provide assistance in doing the procedure.

The staff technologists are responsible for continuously monitoring the performance of the equipment and the technical quality of images produced. Any changes must be communicated to the chief mammography technologist.

1. Technologists must become familiar with the correct operation of the mammography equipment.
2. If the technical quality is unsatisfactory, the technologist must seek a solution to the problem without delay.
3. The procedure should be explained to the patient. When required, the patient's questions should be answered.
4. The patient must be properly positioned to ensure that all the breast tissue is shown.
5. The patient's breast must be adequately compressed.
6. The film must be correctly labeled with the pertinent patient information and the projection performed.
7. The history form should be reviewed with the patient to make sure the correct information is documented.
8. The technician should continue to improve his or her knowledge of the procedure by attending continuing education courses.

Teamwork and communication are the keys to success in mammography. It is imperative to have a reliable level of communication between the chief technologist, the staff technologists, and the radiologists. A technologist who understands the importance of diagnosis of breast disease will try to provide the necessary information for the radiologist. This will ensure that the patient receives the best possible examination.

3.2 The Communication Responsibilities of the Mammographic Technologist

1. Remember that your physical appearance will communicate to the patient the pride you take in your profession and yourself.
2. Greet the patient. Remember to smile and to introduce yourself.
3. Be sensitive to the patient's apprehension. Most apprehension stems from misconceptions about the procedure.
4. Respect the patient's privacy. Be sensitive to how women perceive their own physical appearance.
5. Effective communication will reassure the patient,

giving her comfort and understanding. Create an atmosphere that will help to make this a positive experience.

- Use clear, concise, understandable language to explain the procedure to the patient.
- Use the opportunity, while soliciting information from the patient for the history form, to display concern for the patient's health care.
- Recognize that a breast cancer survivor is often highly educated; thus her anxiety level is high and her needs are different.

6. Recognize that the needs of each patient are different. Know your limitation as a mammographer in providing support and counseling. Refer the patient to the appropriate health care provider.

7. Be responsible for asking questions that provide the information needed to ensure the best possible technical examination; for example, selecting the correct exposure factors or alternative positioning.

8. Explain to the patient when and who will communicate the results of the mammogram. Remind her that if she does not hear from her referring physician, this does not necessarily mean that "All is OK." It is the responsibility of the patient to follow up on her own results.

9. "Do as I say, not as I do" is not the message to give a patient. The mammography technologist must not shun her own responsibilities to herself. Be a role model for the patient.

4. Summary

One of the major disadvantages remaining in mammography today is the rotation of numerous technologists through the mammography room. Lack of interest and experience result in both poor image quality and poor patient care. The technologist's ability to communicate quality, compassion, and consideration will help the patient to relax.

Mammography affords the technologist the opportunity to become more involved with the management of the procedure. Lack of education is still a major hindrance, as most patients are misinformed about mammography. If a woman truly understands the mammography procedure, she will realize that it can save her life by identifying an area of suspicion in a timely fashion. Early detection results in reduced expense and anxiety: fewer severe treatments such as surgery, chemotherapy, or radiation and less emotional stress and anxiety.

6 Techniques in Screen-Film Mammography

Technique as defined by Webster is the "method of accomplishing a desired aim." Often the word *technique* is misinterpreted and is used interchangeably with *exposure factor*. The technique of any radiographic procedure requires an understanding of the entire imaging chain and how it will affect the final outcome of the image. A good technologist will know which factors to alter to obtain a high-quality image.

Before a technologist exposes a patient, the technologist should evaluate the patient and the patient's history form. Knowledge of the mammography equipment, the screen-film combination, the processing environment, and the viewing conditions utilized will aid in correctly exposing the patient to obtain a high-quality examination. In this chapter we discuss the value of compression and its effects on the final image. Also, considerations required to set exposure factors and how to access the final image are discussed.

1. Compression

When screen-film mammography is performed, proper compression is required. *Proper compression* refers to the amount of compression, how it is applied, and its effects on the final image. When minimal compression is applied, the exposure to the pa-

tient is increased, or the patient will pull away from the receptor, resulting in a loss of breast tissue visualized on the final mammogram. An even more detrimental possibility is that a lesion may be missed.

1.1. The Value of Compression

As the compression is applied to the breast, the breast spreads out laterally and the thickness through which the x-ray beam must travel to reach the film is reduced. The breast must be taut to the touch. Compression affects the final image in the following manner (1, 2):

1. Compression reduces exposure or radiation dose to the patient.
2. Compression contributes to improving image quality (Figure 6.1).
   - Compression immobilizes the breast, reducing patient motion.
   - Immobilization of the breast results in additional breast tissue being visualized.
   - Compression permits the parenchymal tissue to be spread, permitting better visualization of the fine architecture.
   - Compression assists in providing close object-to-film distance.
   - Compression provides a uniform thickness of the breast, which results in even penetration and even radiographic density.

43

Whole breast compression

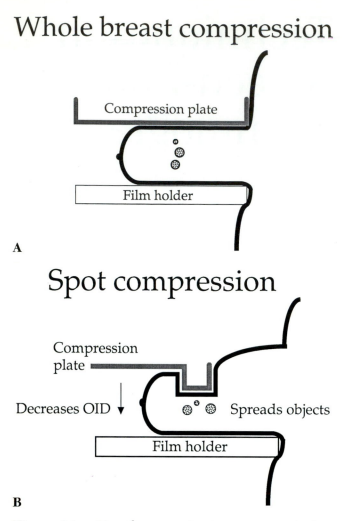

Compression plate

Film holder

A

Spot compression

Compression plate

Decreases OID ↓   Spreads objects

Film holder

B

Figure 6.1. Use of compression in mammography has many advantages(refer to Section 1.1). **A.** Whole-breast compression. **B.** Spot compression helps to further evaluate a suspicious area.

- Reduction of the breast thickness results in a decrease in the scatter radiation, improving subject contrast.

If for any reason the proper amount of compression cannot be applied, this must be documented for the radiologist—that is, on the history form. Some patients are more sensitive to compression than others, etc.

1.2. How to Apply Compression

The most important component to applying compression is the technologist's ability to communicate with the patient. Before starting the procedure, the technologist must tell the patient what to expect. Never use the words *pain* or *hurt* to describe the compression. As discussed in Chapter 5, the patient has often been exposed to the negatives of mammography, and the technologist must attempt to overcome any negative feelings the patient may have.

Some facilities use educational videotapes to educate the patient about the mammographic procedure and what to expect upon entering the examination room. An alternative is to provide literature in the waiting room for the patient to read. Other suggestions to help patients overcome their anxiety are as follows:

1. In the mammography suite, hang a picture or a radiograph of a nonpalpable mass. The radiograph should demonstrate a nonpalpable mass visualized because of compression. The comparison should demonstrate the same mass missed because of poor compression.
2. Hang a poster stating: "We compress because we care." Although many facilities have a poster with this expression, encourage an artistic person to create a unique poster.
3. Educate the referring physicians and their assistants to discuss the mammographic procedure with their patients. Supply the referring physicians with literature for their waiting area(s) or to give to the patients when scheduling them for a mammogram.

Remember, the technologist must communicate with the patient about compression. The more the patient knows or understands about the value of compression, the more she will relax, which makes the technologist's job easier to perform. Some considerations are as follows:

1. Discuss with the patient the importance of compression.
2. Invite the patient to play an active role in applying the compression, allowing her to feel in control. Advise the patient when the compression will be initiated.
3. Apply the compression gradually. Never should the technologist "slam" the compression device down on top of the patient's breast. As compression is applied, the technologist's hand should slide away from the patient and out from under the compression device. When possible, maintain eye contact with the patient. More important, continue to communicate with the patient.
4. The compression must be applied until the breast is taut, but the patient should not experience pain. (*Note:* The technologist must remember that some patients have lower pain thresholds than others.)

5. It is important that the patient feel relaxed. Anxiety produces an increase in physical tension, making the examination more uncomfortable.

Before applying compression, the technologist must consider the *natural mobility of the breast* (Figure 6.2A). The breast is anchored onto the chest from the superior and medial aspects. This means the breast is easier to compress from the inferior and lateral aspects. The technologist must take advantage of this mobility to gain additional breast tissue on the final image. The trick is to "lift" or "move" the breast

before placing it onto the image receptor. If the breast is not lifted properly during the positioning process, the patient may experience discomfort when compression is applied.

1. Craniocaudal view (Figure 6.2B and C): Lift the patient's breast, which will give the breast more "flexibility." Raise the image receptor to the patient carefully. The receptor and the inframammary crease must be so positioned as to obtain as much breast tissue as possible. A receptor that is too high or too low will result in a loss of posterior breast tissue visualized on the mammogram (see Chapter 7, Sections 1.1 and 5.1).
2. Mediolateral oblique view: As you are positioning the patient, push the breast medially. Raise the image receptor to meet the breast. In effect, the image receptor is part of the compression. Once the breast has been pushed medially, lower the compression. If, during the mediolateral oblique view, the patient experiences discomfort due to "pulling" of the breast tissue by the compression device, reposition the patient (see Chapter 7, Sections 1.2 and 5.2).

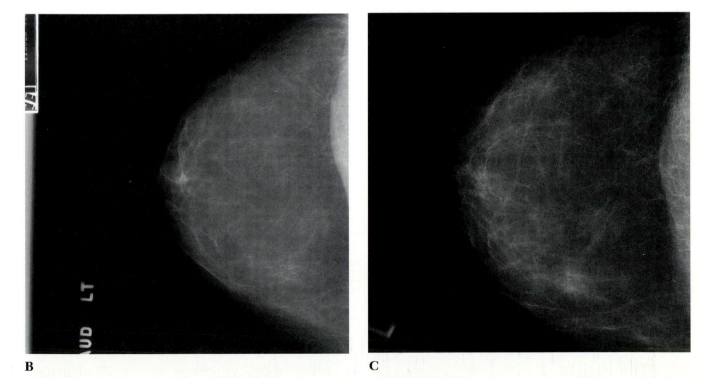

A

B

C

Figure 6.2. Demonstration of the natural mobility of the breast. **A.** The breast is easier to compress from the inferior and the lateral aspect. **B.** Craniocaudal view, improperly positioned. **C.** Properly positioned craniocaudal view, demonstrating more posterior breast tissue.

1.3. What Is the Correct Amount of Compression?

When vigorous compression is applied to the breast, the breast skin will be taut. Some state that compression must be applied until the patient is uncomfortable. Everyone's pain threshold is different. The best method to determine the amount of compression is to feel the breast tissue after compression is applied. Once the patient's skin is taut, compression is adequate.

- For the craniocaudal view, check for tautness on the medial and lateral aspects.
- For the 90° lateral and mediolateral oblique views, check at the superior and posterior aspects of the breast. If the patient reports any discomfort, the technologist must ensure that it is not due to "pinching" of the patient or improper positioning.

2. Exposure Factors

It is the responsibility of the technologist to know how to set the correct exposure factors properly. All too often, technical factors are assumed: "As long as there is a phototimer, nothing else is required." The average patient is usually not a problem. Even when using an automatic exposure control (AEC), an exposure chart must be established.

Selection of exposure factors is affected by several variables:

- the patient
- the mammography equipment
- the screen-film combination
- the processing environment
- the viewing environment

Once all these variables are considered and it is understood how they influence each other, one can better understand how changing each variable may affect the image contrast and perceptible detail.

2.1. The Patient

The patient's history as well as the breast tissue composition and size of the breast will influence the choice of exposure factors. Variables that may affect the exposure factors selected are:

- patient age
- hormone treatment
- implants: saline, silicone
- radiation treatment
- genetics
- breast thickness
- number of births
- surgery: scar tissue, hematoma, tissue removal
- pre- or postmenopausal breast
- lactating breast
- abnormal pathology
- ability to compress

Considerations relating to the variables listed above are as follows:

1. Is the patient on hormone therapy? An older woman who is taking estrogen may require additional exposure, as the hormones may alter the makeup of the breast.
2. Has the patient recently received radiation treatment to the breast? The area that has been treated with radiation may be thicker and more difficult to penetrate.
3. Has the patient recently had breast surgery? A large hematoma or scar tissue may be troublesome. Scar tissue is often thicker than the surrounding breast tissue. Exposure factors should be increased accordingly.
4. What is the patient's age? Has she had children? The older woman who has had multiple full-term pregnancies will usually have adipose breast tissue. It may be necessary to decrease exposure.
5. Is the patient lactating? The breast of a young woman who is nursing is very dense. Exposure factors should be increased, a faster screen-film combination should be used, or a more appropriate target-filtration combination should be selected.
6. Has the patient been diagnosed with some type of breast disease, such as Paget's? Exposure with lower mAs and kVp values should be used if possible.
7. How thick is the breast once compression is applied? Does breast thickness change from the craniocaudal projection to the mediolateral oblique projection?
8. What is the composition of the breast tissue type? Is the tissue adipose or dense? The radiograph of

an adipose breast will appear gray unless alterations are made to the exposure factors.

Before the patient is exposed, the technologist should try to learn as much about her breast history as possible. Techniques should be adjusted accordingly. Some helpful hints are given in Chapter 10.

2.2. Mammography Equipment

Every manufacturer of mammography equipment will suggest the correct exposure factors for its unit. The user's manual should be consulted. The manufacturer should be asked to recommend how exposure factors can be adjusted when necessary. There are several factors that must be kept in mind when establishing technique charts: selection of kVp, mA, time and the target/filtration material. Every facility is unique, and exposure factor charts must be established for each facility involved.

2.2.1. kVp Selection

The kVp, which controls the wavelength of the x-ray beam or the penetrating power, influences subject contrast and exposure latitude, ultimately influencing the image contrast. Selecting the proper kVp requires knowledge of the given breast tissue type(see Section 1.1) and the image recording system. At all times, the kVp that will provide the optimum image should be selected. This depends upon several factors, including the following:

1. The generator type used often determines the image contrast. The kVp recommended by the equipment manufacturer should be used.
2. When the correct equipment calibration is not maintained and performance is not within the tolerances, there may be a loss of contrast or increase in patient exposure.
3. The target material and beam filtration influences the image contrast and the kVp selected. The kVp recommended by the equipment manufacturer should be followed. The suggested kVp ranges are as follows:
   • molybdenum target tube: from 24 to 30 kVp
   • rhodium target tube: from 26 to 32 kVp
   • tungsten target tube: from 22 to 26 kVp
4. Optimize the processing environment for the screen-film combination per the film manufacturer's recommendation.

5. Consideration must be given to the patient's breast tissue structure when selecting the proper kVp value. According to Jenkins (1), "Certain pathology produces an increase or decrease in the radiodensity. This will make the normally accepted kVp for the region unacceptable."

All factors must be considered before selecting the kVp. The mammographer must be aware of the variables and their effect on the final image.

2.2.2. Anode/Filter Selection

Historically altering kVp was the most effective method of altering beam quality for the glandular tissue types. Recent introductions to dual-anode/filter mammography equipment permit the operator additional flexibility in setting exposure factors, especially for glandular and large patient(s). The correct kVp selection for the appropriate target and/or filter recommended by the equipment manufacturer should be used (see Section 2.2.1. for the recommended kVp for the various target materials available). This newer mammography equipment has the ability to automatically select the appropriate kVp and target/filter for the patient (see AEC, section 2.2.6.) based upon the patient breast tissue composition and the compressed breast thickness. Consideration must be given to the fact that often the same kVp will be employed but the x-ray beam will be stronger, thus providing better penetration. The films may demonstrate loss of contrast.

2.2.3. mAs Selection

Some mammography units require adjusting the mAs to alter image density. Increasing the mAs will increase the optical density on the final mammogram. By increasing the mAs, usually the time is most affected. In other words, for a given kVp selected, by increasing the mAs, the mA will remain constant and the length of the exposure will increase. As stated previously, consideration must be given to the reciprocity law failure. With some of the commercially available equipment, as the mAs increases, the dimensions for the electron beam may increase. This will depend on the tube design. As the electron beam increases, so does the potential for a decline in image sharpness.

2.2.4 mA Selection

For a given time and kVp, mA will control the x-ray beam intensity, provided that the kVp selected is optimum for the breast tissue composition and thickness. The mA is used to control film blackening. Mammography equipment may or may not have a variable mA selection. In those units that have variable mA, the technologist should be careful to determine how it will affect the focal spot size.

> **Example:** Equipment X may have a selection of 15, 25, 50, 100, and 150 mA. When the small focal spot is selected for magnification, only 15 mA may be used. When the option is available, an increase in mA will increase the image density or the film will appear darker. A decrease in mA will mean a lighter film. With some of the available mammography equipment, the mA changes with the selected kVp.

If calibration of the equipment is not maintained, the mA will drop or drift out of accepted tolerance levels. If this occurs, the images will be too light or too dark, especially when manual exposures are utilized. An AEC will usually compensate with exposure time.

2.2.5. Exposure Time Selection

Once the proper kVp is selected for the breast tissue type, the exposure time is often the only method that can be used to control the image density. The exposure timer will determine the time an object is exposed to radiation. The length of the exposure must always be a consideration in mammography because of the reciprocity law failure (see Chapter 4, Section 2.5).

Some mammography machines are limited by low output. The exposure time is the major factor to affect image density. Unfortunately, longer exposure times may result in lack of image sharpness due to patient motion. In such a situation, it is helpful to have several different speed screens available. If patient motion is not a problem, increasing the exposure time will increase image density; that is, the film will appear darker.

2.2.6. Automatic Exposure Control

Most mammography today is performed with the aid of an AEC device. Once the kVp is set, breast thickness and breast tissue are compensated for by adjusting the mAs. Density control knobs are available to increase or decrease exposure density. The operator's manual should be consulted for the correct operation of the particular piece of equipment.

Several newer mammography units have the ability to select the kVp, target, and/or filtration material independent of the operator. Once the patient has been positioned correctly and the breast compressed, based upon a preexposure measurement, the AEC has an automatic exposure factor selection mechanism which chooses the appropriate kVp, the target, and/or filtration.

Some of the older mammography machines do not have the ability to "track" with the various breast thicknesses. Many older units can be upgraded. The equipment manufacturer should be consulted. Prepare an exposure technique chart when exposure density must be altered.

One other consideration that must be kept in mind is that most units have a variable-position detector having two or three positions. The detector may be positioned at the chest wall, the body of the breast, or the anterior breast. The placement of the detector will vary with the different breast sizes or for breast tissue composition.

> **Example:** *For an extremely small patient:* the anterior position may miss the breast tissue altogether. This will result in a light film.
> *For an extremely large, glandular patient:* the chest wall position may not be centered to the middle of the patient's breast or to the glandular tissue.

Occasionally, variations in exposure density will occur when using an AEC. One must consider the following:

1. Different-speed screens
2. Screens the same speed but a different life span
3. Screen the same speed but a different batch number
4. Film placed into the cassette incorrectly
5. Incorrect film
6. Correct film but a different batch number
7. Cassette placed into holder incorrectly or upside down
8. AEC's inability to track for breast thickness
9. Inability to consistently position the patient's breast correctly (Figure 6.3)
10. Inability to consistently compress the breast from one projection to another

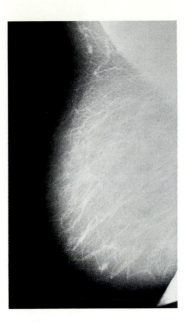

Figure 6.3. Improper penetration, compression, and positioning.

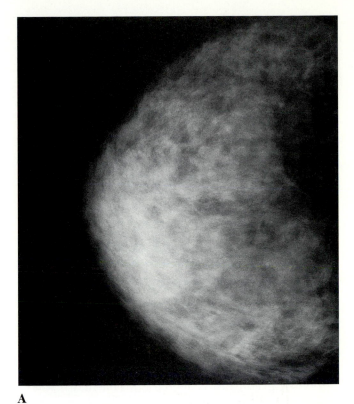

A

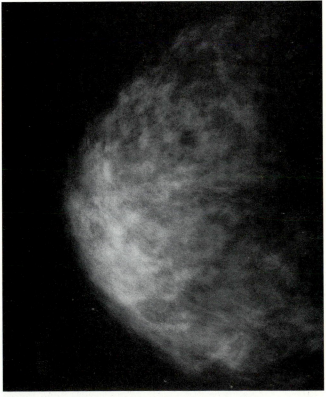

B

Figure 6.4. Placement of the AEC detector. **A.** Craniocaudal view with incorrect placement of the AEC detector. **B.** Correct placement of the AEC detector of the same patient demonstrates correct penetration of the glandular tissue.

11. Fluctuation of density, especially with shorter exposure times
12. Incorrect position of the detector
13. Incorrect selection of anode and/or filtration material.
    - Whenever possible, the detector should be placed under the glandular portion of the breast (Figure 6.4).
    - To determine the correct position of the detector, either the previous films should be looked at, the breast should be palpated, the patient history should be reviewed, or the first film should be checked.

2.2.7. Collimation

Collimation, or restriction of the x-ray beam to a small area, reduces scattered radiation, enhancing image contrast. When the entire film format is exposed, the image may appear "darker" than a spot-coned view. When collimating to a very small area of the breast, the technologist must increase exposure. To maintain a constant density, the exposure should be increased by 25 to 35%. The exposure should be altered with mAs instead of kVp so that subject contrast remains the same.

2.3. Screen-Film Combination

No two films are alike in their response to exposure. As the trend in mammography goes more in the direction of high contrast, the technologist must realize that the faster and/or higher in contrast the screen-film combination, the less exposure latitude the technologist has to select. This means the technologist must consider the entire imaging chain before exposing the patient and keep several factors in mind (1):

1. Film latitude is the ability of a film to respond to a range of exposures and record them as useful densities.
2. The faster the screen-film system, the less the exposure latitude. The less the exposure latitude, the less number of choices available when selecting exposure factors.
3. To give a film more exposure latitude, one may select a higher kVp. Unfortunately, when this is done, the contrast is decreased. This may result in the loss of information.
4. A dense breast contains tissue that is high in contrast. When this type of patient is exposed, exposure latitude is often minimal.
5. Exposure latitude depends on the breast tissue type and the kVp selected.
6. An object low in contrast, such as an adipose breast, will appear to have a long range of exposure latitude.

2.4. Processing Conditions

The quality of the mammography image is influenced by the processing conditions.

> **Example:** Processing a film at a lower-than-recommended developer temperature may result in more exposure latitude or reduce the contrast of the final image.

Some film types perform better in extended processing cycles. The added time in the developer increases the contrast and the speed of the film. Exposure factors must be established when going to extended processing, especially when the film responds to the longer cycle. Usually the strength of the processing solutions is overlooked (Figure 6.5A and B). In mammography, it is preferable to use a highly active chemical system. Too often large quantities of chemical solutions are put into a large holding tank. When fresh solutions are added to the holding tank, technologists can use "normal" exposure factors. Over the course of the month, technologists must increase exposure factors to maintain a constant image density and to compensate for the aging or dilution of the chemicals. The processor should be

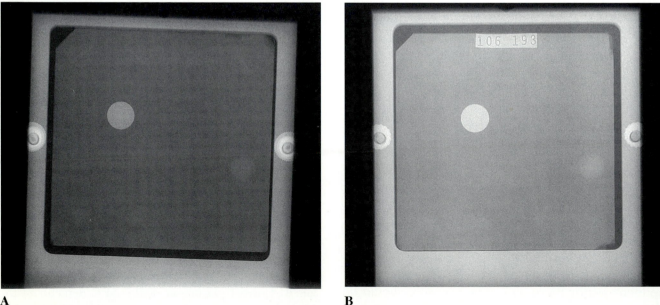

A   B

Figure 6.5. The effects of chemistry on the final image. **A.** The film manufacturers recommendations have been followed. **B.** The film is underdeveloped.

stabilized and monitored to minimize the need to increase exposure to the patient.

2.5. Viewing Environment

A poor viewing environment will efface or obliterate many advantages of even the most optimum image quality. Proper viewing conditions are defined as (a) view boxes that produce a minimum of 3500 nit, (b) masking of the mammograms (black cardboard, black film, or special view boxes with inherent masking capabilities), and (c) minimize the ambient light by turning off the overhead lights, turning out the view boxes not in use, closing the drapes on window(s) (Chapter 9, Sections 5.11 and 10).

A proper viewing environment includes not only an optimal area for evaluating the mammographic image but a locality where extraneous distractions (interruptions, noise, etc.) are minimal.

3. Operator-Controlled Factors

Up until now the key factors that influence the final image have been discussed, but independently of each other. For a given imaging chain and a given pa-

tient, how are the exposure factors altered? How will selecting the proper kVp, anode/filter, and mAs influence image contrast and perceptible detail?

Until recently, in practical applications, the technologist could alter exposure factors with only two variables: (1) the mAs and (2) the kVp. Variation of these and anode/filter affect x-ray intensity and image density. Knowing which factor to alter is sometimes tricky. If a change is made, which one should be selected? When an AEC is used, this decision is made automatically unless the patient's breast tissue is not within "normal" limits. In mammography, the best rule to follow is this: select the proper anode/filter and/or kVp for the breast tissue type. Compensate to alter the image density with mAs.

3.1. How Does mAs Affect the Image?

An image may be (1) too dark, (2) too light (Figure 6.6A), or (3) properly exposed (Figure 6.6B). The mAs may be used to control the average image density.

1. An overexposed image is usually too dark. Selecting an mAs too high for the breast tissue type will mean a loss of perceptible detail. The light areas or the "whites" will also be overexposed, or too dark.
2. An underexposed image is usually too light. The selected mAs for a given breast tissue type is too

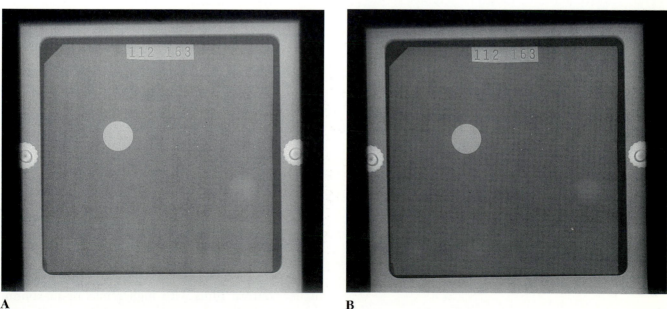

A   **B**

Figure 6.6. The effects of altering mAs on film. **A.** The phantom image is too light. **B.** Properly exposed phantom image.

low, thus there may be a loss of diagnostic information.

3. Selecting the proper mAs for the breast provides an image with the correct density. The properly exposed image will have maximum information—the most visible information; more importantly, it will be a diagnostic-quality radiograph with perceptible detail.

3.2.   How Does kVp Affect the Image?

The kVp is changed when it becomes necessary to alter image contrast. The kVp controls the spectrum of the x-ray beam, which varies the penetrating power of the radiation, which in turn alters the subject contrast. If a kVp is too high for the breast tissue type selected, the image will lose contrast. The image may appear too dark or gray, which results in a loss of image contrast and loss of the perceived detail. An image with a kVp that is too low (Figure 6.7A), even slightly too low, will have high contrast in the medium densities. The overall appearance of the image, however, will result in a loss of detail in the dense breast tissue. The correct kVp (Figure 6.7B) not only provides good image contrast but the optimum per-

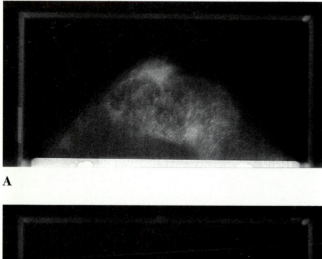

A

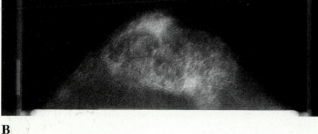

B

Figure 6.7. Increasing kVp gives one the impression that the image is darker. **A.** Increased kVp reduces the contrast and perceived detail. **B.** Correct kVp selected.

ceived detail over the entire density range within the breast tissue. A properly exposed film provides the radiologist with a diagnostic film with the required information.

3.3.   How Does the Anode/Filter Affect the Image?

The anode/filter are changed when it becomes necessary to increase the penetration power of the radiation (Figure 6.8). Altering the anode/filter combination improperly may result in a loss of image contrast and perceived detail. It is important for the operator to correctly select the appropriate anode/filter for the patient's breast tissue type.

For example, in selecting a rhodium/rhodium combination for the average 50/50 breast tissue type, the image may appear flat or gray and appear to have lost contrast and detail. Or, conversely, for the young, glandular breast-tissue type, the image will appear properly exposed and the glandular tissue will be penetrated.

4.   What Determines Adequate Exposure?

The final image or the "look" of the mammogram must be determined by the facility's radiologist. When accessing the final image, it is imperative to obtain the best image visualizing the important elements of the breast.

The following are guidelines/recommendations for adequate exposure on the final image:

1. The desired optical density in the main glandular area should be 1.3 to 1.5.
2. The optical density in the most glandular areas should be no less than 0.7.
3. The skin area should have an optical density of 3.0.

Note: These recommendations are just that and depend upon the total imaging chain.

A subject of much discussion is the need for higher-contrast films with high Dmax or maximum density, as well as the significance of the visualization of skin line. Sometimes abnormalities are seen just below the skin line. Therefore if the skin line is not

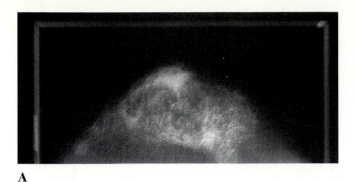
A

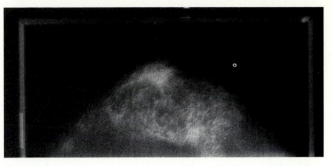
B

Figure 6.8. The effects of anode/filter variation. **A.** Molybdenum/molybdenum combination. **B.** Rhodium/rhodium combination.

visualized, a subtle abnormality may be missed. As a rule, it is preferred to penetrate the glandular tissue properly as opposed to visualizing the skin line. If subcutaneous lesions are suspected, it is not difficult to take a second image.

If visualization of skin line is the objective, it is appropriate to consider several alternatives:

1. The film sensitometric response characteristics. The technologist has the least control of the film design.
2. Proper viewing conditions and masking. If correct viewing conditions are utilized, the skin line will be visualized most of the time. (See Section 1.5 and Chapter 9, Section 5.11 or 10.)
3. Increasing kVp is one acceptable method to try and achieve skin line. This, however, does decrease subject contrast and may compromise image contrast.
4. Reducing mAs to lower overall average image density, the technique employed in tangential views for skin calcifications, will improve the skin line visibility while lowering exposure to the patient. The pitfall of lowering the mAs may be the non-visualization of breast parenchymal patterns.

At no time may radiographic techniques be compromised potentially losing the early signs of carcinoma. If necessary, especially if the skin line is an area of question and concern, expose one view with altered exposure factors.

Sometimes, after an image is evaluated, it may be beneficial to alter exposure factors intentionally to further analyze an area in question. In soft-tissue imaging, such as that of the breast, the density differences between the various structures are subtle. Consideration of the entire imaging chain, the patient's history, and selection of the proper exposure factors for the patient to provide the optimum image is critical.

5. Correctly Labeling the Mammographic Image

All radiographic films are permanent documents and must include unique patient identification data exposed (flashed) onto the film. This is no different in mammography.

As demonstrated in Figure 6.9, all information must be visualized, but away from the breast tissue. The projection labels, to include labeling the side of the patient visualized, must be placed close to the axillary region of the breast tissue.

The required permanent labeling must include the following:

1. The facility's name, the facility's address, the patient name (first, middle initial, and last), the patient x-ray number (or unique identification system or number), and the date the procedure is performed. These are exposed onto the film electronically or with an identification camera.
2. The projection performed (for example, CC or MLO) and the side of the patient visualized (for example, R or L). These are exposed onto the film electronically or markers are placed onto the image receptor.
3. The technologist's initials or identification number who performed the examination. The technologist's initials/ID can be written onto the film with a felt-tip marker, or, preferably, each tech-

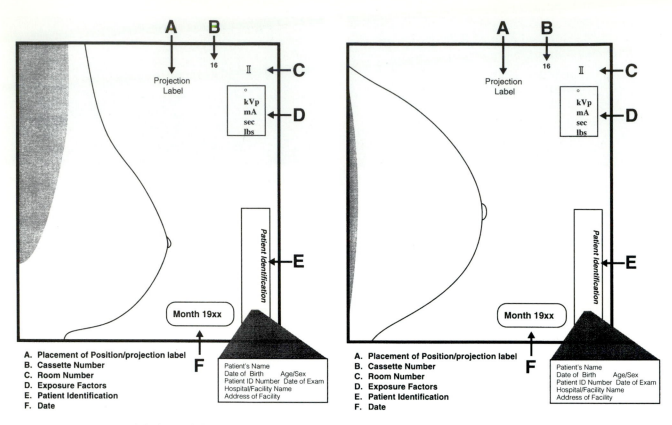

Figure 6.9. Correct labeling of the mammography film(s).

nologist will have an ID system, such as a marker, that is exposed onto the final image.

4. Cassette and screen number (see Chapter 9, Section 5.6, on how to correctly identify cassettes and screens).

Additionally, it is strongly recommended the final image include the following:

1. Date stickers.
2. Exposure factors (either by permanent electronic digital ID system or by self-adhesive sticker).
3. Dedicated mammography unit number or room number.

6. Evaluating the Final Image

Before the radiographs are submitted to the radiologist for final approval, it is the responsibility of the technologist to critique the images. A technologist newly transferred into the mammography department must be taught what a good mammogram looks like. The technologist must be taught how to achieve the image quality that the radiologist is looking for in the images that he or she is presented with.

The technologist should be told how much responsibility she or he has during the procedure. For example, if additional views are necessary, does the technologist have permission to take the extra views without discussing it with the radiologist? It is especially important to establish what responsibility a technologist does have when immediate supervision by a radiologist is unavailable.

Whenever possible, the films from the preceding mammograms should be available before the patient is exposed. The technologist should review the images and take note of any changes that would improve the image quality from the previous year. If the patient is having her first baseline examination, it is helpful to have the first image checked before the remaining routine views are completed. Document the exposure factors on the patient films for future reference.

The previous films are important not only for the technologist to view before exposing the patient but also for the radiologist to review. A patient's previous films are like a history book. Reference films permit the radiologist to follow a suspicious area or detect any parenchymal changes as soon as possible.

When the routine views are completed, the technologist should document any difficulties that may have arisen during performance of the examination. For example, if the technologist did not feel that she or he could apply vigorous compression, this should be documented. Also, the technologist should review the routine images to determine whether additional views are necessary. If so, the technologist should proceed with the extra projections.

Once the technologist has completed the procedure and before presenting them to the radiologist, she or he should evaluate the radiographs thoroughly for the following:

1. Is the patient properly positioned? The radiographs should include the area of clinical suspicion.
2. Are the images properly penetrated? If a dense area is seen in the breast, has action been taken to better visualize that area?
3. Are the films properly labeled with all the pertinent patient information?
4. Are the images free of artifacts? Artifacts can be multiple. Check for the following:
   • deodorant or powders (see Figure 6.10)
   • processor artifacts
   • handling artifacts
   • patient anatomic artifacts (such as a chin superimposed over the breast—Figure 6.11)
   • dust or dirt

• equipment failure related problems
• patient motion

Upon presenting the patient's portfolio to the radiologist, the technologist should be prepared to discuss the patient and the images with the radiologist. In those facilities where a radiologist is not available, the final evaluation of the images is critical. At all times, the technologist should try to make the patient feel comfortable and confident that she has received the best possible examination. The patient should be informed of what to expect once she has left the mammography department, including a possible request for a return visit for additional views.

7. Summary

The correct technique for performing mammography is more than just turning on the mammography equipment and positioning the patient (Figure 6.12). Technique is taking the entire imaging chain into consideration to properly produce a quality mammogram. As pointed out in previous chapters, each patient and each facility is different. Every mammogram must be tailored to the patient.

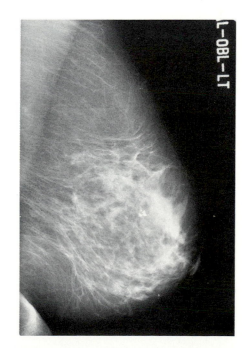

Figure 6.11. Patient's chin radiographed onto the final image due to poor positioning.

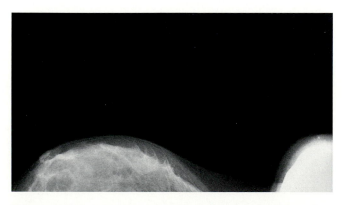

Figure 6.10. Patient with deodorant or powder on her breast. Note the "microcalcification" appearance on the radiograph.

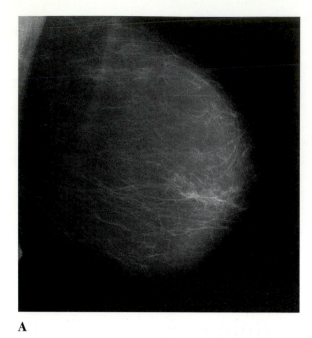

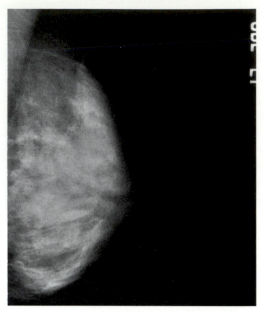

A   B

Figure 6.12.   Proper positioning and adjustment of exposure factors are required in order to achieve the optimal image for each breast type. **A.** Patient with adipose breast tissue. **B.** Patient with glandular breast tissue.

References

1. Jenkins D. Radiographic Photography and Imaging Processes. Baltimore: University Park Press; 1980:28–29, 91–109.
2. Logan WW. Screen film mammography technique: Compression and other factors, in *Reduced Dose Mammography:* New York: Masson; 1979:418–419.
3. American College of Radiology Committee on Quality Assurance in Mammography: Mammography Quality Control, Reston, VA: American College of Radiology; 1994.
4. Ecklund GW, Cardenosa G. The Art of mammographic positioning. Radiol Clin North Am 1992:3(1):21-53.
5. National Council on Radiation Protection and Measurements. Mammography: A User's Guide. Bethesda, MD: NCRP no. 85; 1986:18-22.

7

Positioning

Mammography produces a detailed radiograph or map of the breast. It is important to define or visualize the small architectural differences between the various structures. Every patient's build is different; thus the mammogram must be tailored to the needs of the individual. Before the patient is exposed radiographically, her habitus or body build (Figure 7.1A) and medical history should be assessed. Any scars, moles, or abnormalities must be noted on the history form. Notations about the patient's breast may be made by visually dividing each breast into quadrants or describing the area on the breast in relation to the face of a clock (Figure 7.1B). If available, the patient's previous films should be checked.

It is imperative, especially when the patient is having the first mammogram, to describe the procedure. When the patient is *anxious*, physical tension may result in an uncomfortable examination. A *relaxed* patient will cooperate, making the procedure easier to perform. When positioning a patient for a mammogram, the technologist must demonstrate as much as possible of the breast tissue on the final image. Three factors must be kept in mind while positioning a patient (1). They are as follows:

1. The patient's chest wall is curved, and the image receptor that is placed against the chest wall has a straight edge.
2. Most breast cancers are found in the upper outer quadrant (Figure 7.2).
3. One must take into consideration the *natural mobility of the patients's breast* (refer to Chapter 6, Section 1.2).

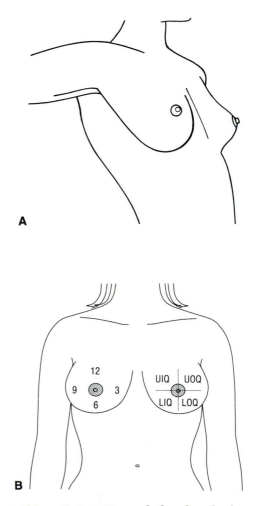

A

B

Figure 7.1. Orientation of the female breast. **A.** Silhouette of chest. Each patient's build is different. **B.** Frontal view of chest. When trying to localize an area of interest, the patient's breast may be described as the face of a clock, or it may be divided into quadrants.

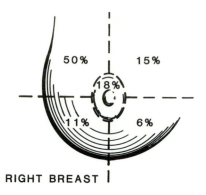

Figure 7.2. Location and frequency of breast cancers.

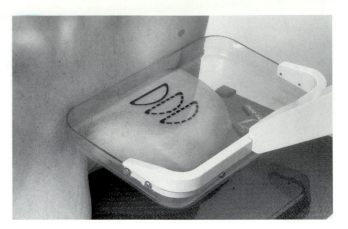

Figure 7.3. Properly positioned craniocaudal view demonstrating the medial aspect of the breast.

The material in this chapter demonstrates positioning. The standard projections are discussed. Adjunctive views may be required to further demonstrate a suspicious lesion. The patient's build may require supplementing the standard views. Problems often encountered in positioning the patient are discussed.

1. Standard Positioning

The most commonly utilized views are the craniocaudal view and the mediolateral oblique projection. These views are discussed.

1.1. Craniocaudal (CC) Projection

The technologist must always try to include as much of the breast tissue as possible. The medial juxtathoracic area, the breast tissue located deep along the chest wall, may be missed when the mediolateral oblique view is made (1). Thus, the technologist must demonstrate the medial aspect of the breast in the craniocaudal view (Figure 7.3). As much of the lateral tissue as possible must be visualized also. The technologist should obtain an exaggerated craniocaudal view when more lateral tissue must be visualized (refer to Section 2.3).

The technologist should begin positioning the patient for this view by standing on the contralateral side or the side opposite of the breast being imaged. In this way the technologist has a better sense of how high to bring the image receptor after lifting the breast and can also maintain eye contact with the patient.

Position of the x-ray tube assembly:

1. The x-ray tube assembly should be positioned such that the central ray is directed from the superior to the inferior aspect of the breast.
2. The C-arm angle should be 0°.

Position of the patient:

1. The patient should be facing the image receptor (which holds the film) of the mammography machine.
2. The patient should be erect (sitting or standing).
3. The outer edge of the image receptor must be firm against the patient's chest wall.
4. The patient's head should be turned away and forward from the side being examined
5. The patient should lean into the receptor.
6. The patient should hold onto the handlebar with the hand of the side not being imaged.

Position of the part (Figure 7.4):

1. Taking advantage of the natural mobility of the breast (see Chapter 6, Section 1.2), the breast should be lifted on top of the image receptor. Elevate the inframammary fold.

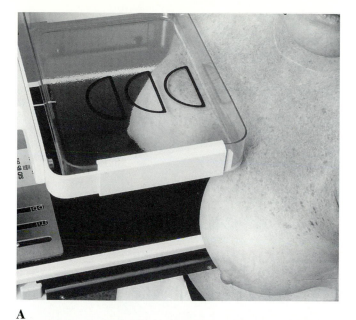

A

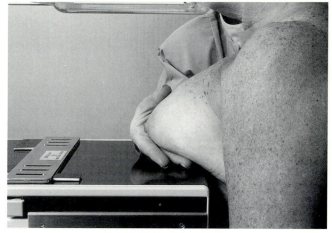

Figure 7.6. Positioning of the craniocaudal view. Lift the breast "up onto" the image receptor.

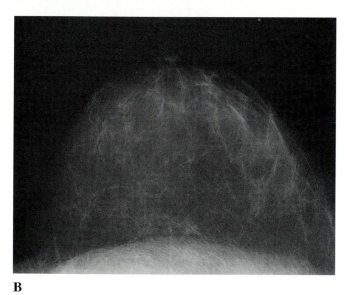

B

Figure 7.4. **A.** Proper positioning of the craniocaudal view. **B.** Craniocaudal view.

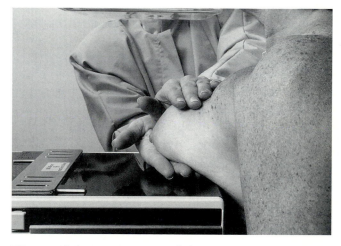

Figure 7.7. Positioning of the CC view. Anchor the breast with both hands, bringing the breast onto the image receptor.

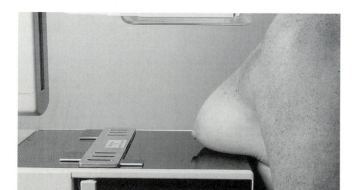

Figure 7.5. The height of the image receptor should be adjusted so the inferior breast surface lies comfortably upon it. Consideration must be given to the natural mobility of the breast.

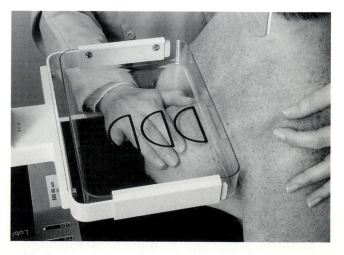

Figure 7.8. Positioning of the CC view. Hold the breast in position while applying final compression.

2. The height of the image receptor should be adjusted so the inferior breast surface lies comfortably upon it (Figure 7.5).

3. Lift the breast up onto the image receptor (Figure 7.6).

4. The posterior breast tissue should be pulled forward. It is strongly recommended that the technologist use both hands to pull the breast "up and out" onto the image receptor (Figure 7.7).

5. The breast must be perpendicular to the chest wall. The breast should be positioned with the nipple in profile and centered on the image receptor.

6. The height of the receptor should be checked from *both* the medial and the lateral aspects of the breast.

7. The breast should be held in position while applying compression (Figure 7.8). The technologist should slowly slide her or his hand away from the chest wall as the compression device is lowered.

8. Care must be taken to place the medial portion of the breast (refer to Figure 7.4A) on top of the receptor. (Visualization of the medial breast tissue is improved by placing the opposite breast over the corner of the image receptor.)

9. Compression should be applied until the lateral and medial borders are taut and the skin firm.

10. Once compression is applied, the patient's arm should hang relaxed at her side with the hand externally rotated.

11. The patient should be instructed to hold still and hold her breath. Then the exposure should begin.

1.2. Mediolateral Oblique (MLO) Projection

The MLO is the most common lateral view utilized in mammography. It allows visualization of the deep structures in the upper outer quadrant of the breast. Unless the patient's anatomy is otherwise, the MLO projection (Figure 7.9A and B) enables more breast tissue to be visualized compared to the 90° mediolateral view. *Note:* In countries using only one view, the MLO is the view of choice.

Position of the x-ray tube assembly:

1. The C arm or the x-ray tube assembly should be rotated such that the image receptor is parallel to the patient's pectoral muscle (Figure 7.10A and B).

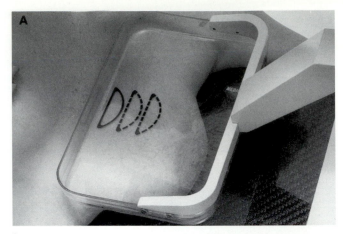

A

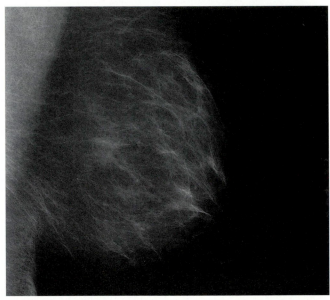

B

Figure 7.9. **A.** Proper positioning of the mediolateral view. **B.** Mediolateral view.

2. The angle of the C arm is usually 30 to 60°. *Note:* Patients' body habitus will vary, thus requiring the angle on the C arm to be adjusted to each patient's build. For example, the tall, thin patient will have more of a vertical orientation, whereas the short, stocky patient may require a greater angle.

Central ray:

1. The central ray should be directed from the superior medial to the inferior lateral aspect of the breast.

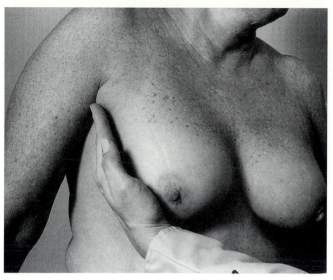

A

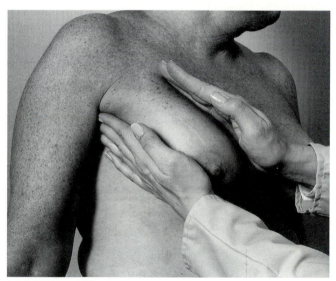

B

Figure 7.10.   A and B. Properly determine the angle for the mediolateral oblique view.

2. The central ray should be directed approximately at the level of the nipple.

Position of the patient:

1. The patient should be erect.
2. The patient should be facing the mammography machine with the image receptor along the lateral side.
3. It is helpful to have the patient's affected hip aligned with the bottom of the image receptor.

Care must be taken so that the patient does not approach the bucky which results in her standing behind the bucky. This will result in lost breast tissue on top of the bucky; the lower posterior breast tissue will not be imaged on the film (Figure 7.11).

4. It is advantageous to have the patient bend at the waist and lean into the mammography unit. This is especially beneficial for those patients who are thick around the middle.
5. The patient's arm should rest along the top of the image receptor. Care must be taken to ensure that the latissimus is placed along the chest-wall edge of the image receptor, not on top of the image receptor (Figure 7.12A and B).
6. With the patient aligned with the image receptor along the lateral side, the image receptor should be positioned parallel to the pectoral muscle. The angle will vary from 30 to 60°, measured from the vertical. Position the pectoral muscle parallel to the image receptor.

> **Suggestion:**   A tall vertical patient closer to 90°. The short horizontal patient closer to 30°.

Position of the part:

1. The breast should be placed on top of the image receptor in the mediolateral projection with the lateral aspect of the breast on the image receptor and the nipple in profile (Figure 7.12 A and B). As described in Chapter 6, Section 1.2, lift the breast medially using the natural mobility of the breast to maximize the amount of breast tissue visualized.

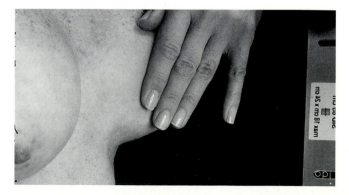

Figure 7.11.   The inframammary crease must be included on the final image.

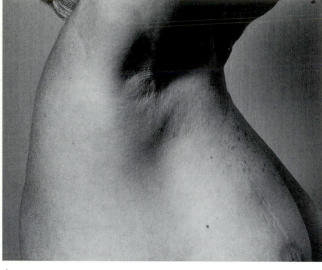

A

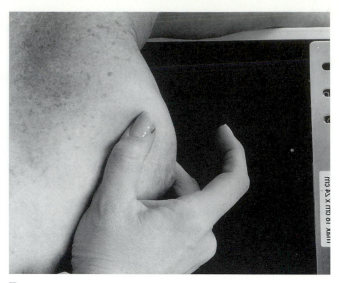

B

Figure 7.12. **A.** The latissimus dorsi is placed along the chest-wall edge of the image receptor, not in front of the receptor.

B. The patient's arm should rest along the top of the image receptor. Initial lifting of the breast onto the image receptor.

2. Care should be taken to include the axillary tail, pectoral muscle, and inframammary crease.
3. The breast should be pulled away from the chest wall. (*Note:* The breast must not drop but must be pulled up, out, and away from the chest wall.) (Figure 7.13.)
4. Compression should be applied.
   - The compression device should skim the sternum parallel to the pectoral muscle.
   - The upper outer edge of the compression device should be positioned right under or skim the clavicle.
   - The compression must be taut.
5. The compression should be checked by feeling the superior and inferior edges of the breast.
6. When necessary, the patient should hold her opposite breast out of the way.
7. Before exposure is initiated, the patient should hold her breath.

1.3 Image Evaluation

After taking the two routine views, the technologist can "double check" to be sure enough of the breast tissue is visualized on the mammogram. Using a ruler or tape measure, take measurements from the nipple to the edge of the film. The craniocaudal view should include, within 1 cm, the amount of tissue measured on the mediolateral oblique view.

2. Additional Views (Supplemental)

Supplemental projections become useful when the standard views selected are inadequate. Sometimes patient history or body build is such that the stan-

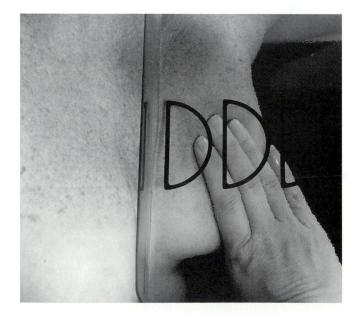

Figure 7.13. The breast is pulled up, out, and away from the chest wall. The breast is held in position while the compression is applied.

dard projections are difficult to obtain. Other reasons for taking additional views are as follows (2, 3):

1. Additional views become necessary when a suspicious area is seen in one of the routine views but not on the second projection.
2. Additional views may allow the patient to avoid the trauma of having an invasive procedure such as a needle localization.
3. Additional views are necessary when other tissue is superimposed on a suspicious area.

When a lesion is superimposed on top of dense breast tissue, the following should be tried (1):

1. If the lesion or mass is large, take the supplemental views at a large angle from the standard views. For example, craniocaudal versus oblique versus lateral.
2. If the area of interest is small, take additional views at small angle increments (plus or minus 5 to 10°) from the routine views. For example, the rolled views.

Although many of the additional views appear very similar, each has its own value. The technologist should select the view most useful to make an accurate diagnosis. Before taking additional views, the technologist should explain the situation to the patient so as to alleviate anxiety.

2.1. 90° Lateral Projection(s)

The contact lateral (straight lateral, or 90° lateral) view may be performed in the lateral-to-medial projection or medial-to-lateral projection. The mediolateral projection can be used as the second view or can be used to complement the existing views taken. The 90° lateral view is used whenever it is necessary to take two images that are perpendicular to each other, as, for example, before a needle localization. A straight lateral view is also advantageous when it is necessary to demonstrate air-fluid-fat levels or "teacup" type calcifications.

2.1.1. Mediolateral (ML) Projection (Figure 7.14A and B)

Position of the x-ray tube assembly:

1. The x-ray tube assembly is rotated to the horizontal position 90° off the 0° angle.

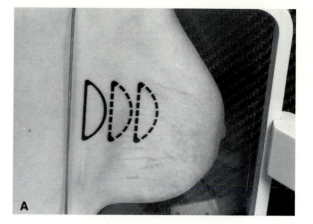

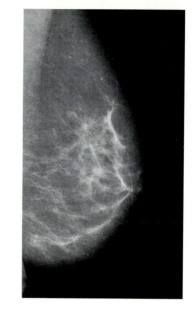

Figure 7.14. **A.** Proper positioning of the mediolateral view. **B.** Mediolateral view.

2. The C-arm configuration is raised until the patient's arm rests on the top of the image receptor. The breast must be centered to the image receptor.

Central ray:

1. The central ray should be directed from the medial to the lateral aspect of the breast.
2. The central ray should be directed to the center of the breast at the chest wall.

Position of the patient:

1. The patient should be erect and facing the mammography machine.
2. The arm should rest on top of the image receptor.

Position of the part:

1. The lateral aspect of the breast should be against the image receptor.
2. The breast should be positioned such that it is centered to the image receptor.
3. The breast should be pulled up and away from the chest wall.
4. The nipple should be in profile.
5. While the breast is held in position, compression should be applied until the tissue is taut. The compression device should skim the sternum.
6. The patient should hold the opposite breast back away from the breast being radiographed.
7. Compression should be completed, and the patient should be asked to hold her breath until the exposure is completed.

2.1.2. Lateromedial (LM) Projection (Figure 7.15)

The lateromedial view is often used to (1) improve the detail of a lesion located in the medial aspect of the breast or (2) perform preoperative localization of an inferior and/or lateral lesion. Some patients' builds require the lateromedial view to demonstrate the medial breast tissue. The lateromedial view may be more comfortable for these patients.

Position of the x-ray tube assembly:

The x-ray tube assembly should be rotated 90°.

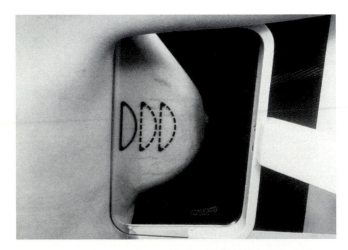

Figure 7.15. **A.** Proper positioning of the lateromedial view.

Central ray:

The central ray should be directed from the lateral to the medial aspect of the breast.

Position of the patient:

1. The patient should face the image receptor.
2. The patient's sternum should rest along the chest wall edge (or slightly offset toward the radiographed breast) of the image receptor.
3. The patient's arm of the side being examined should be placed on top of the handlebars. The arm should not be lifted straight up over the head. When this is done the breast is pulled away from the image receptor.

Position of the part:

1. The medial aspect of the breast should be placed against the center of the image receptor (Figure 7.15).
2. The breast should be lifted up and over onto the receptor.
3. It may be necessary to rotate the patient into the receptor until the nipple is in profile.
4. The compression device should skim the rib cage. Compression should be applied until the breast tissue is taut.

2.2. Caudocranial (FB, or From Below) Projection

The caudocranial or reverse CC view is helpful in the following cases:

1. If the patient has a lesion in the superior or upper quadrants of the breast, the caudocranial view may improve resolution.
2. If the patient is small or a muscular male; it is easier to compress the inferior portion of the breast (Figure 7.16A and B).
3. The patient is kyphotic or has a pacemaker.
4. A needle localization is performed from the inferior aspect of the breast so that there is easier access to a lesion located in the lower quadrants of the breast.

Positioning of the x-ray tube assembly:

1. The x-ray tube assembly should be rotated 180°: that is, it should be upside down.
2. The image receptor should be against the chest wall superior to the breast.

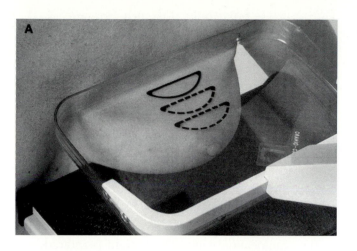

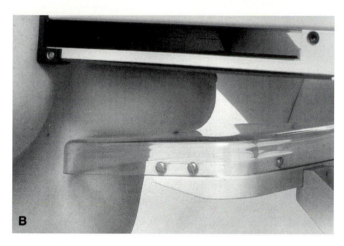

Figure 7.16. **A.** Proper positioning of the craniocaudal view of a small patient. **B.** Positioning of the caudocranial view of the same patient to visualize more breast tissue.

Position of the patient:

1. The patient should face the mammography unit.
2. The patient should be erect.

Position of the part:

1. The breast should be positioned with the superior surface of the breast centered to the image receptor.
2. While the breast is compressed, it is important to hold the breast up and in position.
3. The nipple should be in profile.
4. Care must be taken to make sure abdominal tissue does not interfere with or superimpose on the breast tissue.
5. Once the breast is compressed, the medial and lateral surfaces should be checked for tautness.

2.3. Exaggerated Craniocaudal Projection (XCCL)

The exaggerated craniocaudal projection or the rotated craniocaudal view helps to visualize the lateral aspect of the breast, which may not be radiographed in the standard craniocaudal view. Other situations in which the rotated craniocaudal view is advantageous include the following (2, 3):

1. The patient is obese and the breast tissue extends to the lateral chest wall, or the breast "wraps" around the patient's chest.
   or
2. A lesion is seen in the oblique projection but not in the craniocaudal view.

Position of the x-ray tube assembly:

1. The x-ray tube assembly should be angled 5° into the lateral aspect of the breast (Figure 7.17A through C).
   or
2. Some technologists prefer to rotate the patient to emphasize the lateral portion of the breast. The C arm should be 0°.

Central ray:

1. The central ray should be directed 5° from the superior to the inferior lateral aspect of the breast.
2. The central ray should be directed between the nipple and the lateral breast tissue.

Position of the patient:

1. The patient should face the mammography unit.
2. The patient should be in a position similar to the craniocaudal projection.

Position of the part:

1. The patient's breast should be positioned as in the craniocaudal projection (see Section 1.1).
2. Turn the patient such that the lateral and posterior breast tissue is placed on top of the image receptor.
3. If the patient is relaxed, the lateral breast tissue is easier to position.
4. The breast should be held in position until compression is applied.

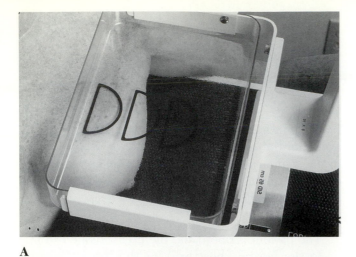

A

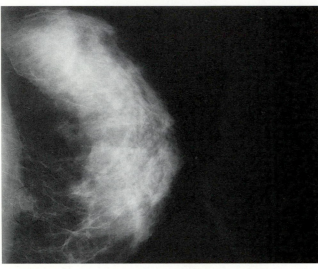

B

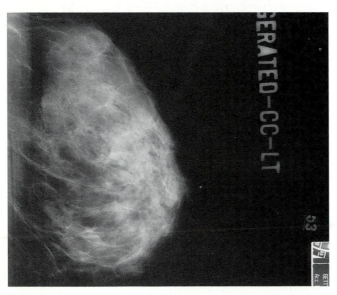

C

Figure 7.17. **A**. Proper positioning of the exaggerated craniocaudal view emphasizing the lateral aspect of the breast. After taking the craniocaudal view (**B**), it may be necessary to take an exaggerated craniocaudal view (**C**) to visualize additional lateral breast tissue.

2.4. Axillary Tail (AT) View

The axillary tail view (formerly known as the Cleopatra view or sometimes as the focal compression oblique view of the axillary tail) is beneficial when trying to visualize the "tail" of the breast (Figure 7.18A through E) and can be performed in one of two ways:

1. The x-ray tube is rotated (a) for the patient who has difficulty lying back onto the image receptor, or (b) for the technologist who prefers this method of positioning.
or
2. The image receptor remains in the position as for the craniocaudal view. The patient is rotated.

(*Note:* The first projection is the most comfortable for the patient.)

Position of the x-ray tube assembly:

1. The x-ray tube assembly should be rotated from 10 to 30° from the superior medial to the inferior lateral aspect of the breast.
or
2. The x-ray equipment should remain at a 0° angle.

Position of the patient:

1. The patient should be erect with the image receptor along the side being examined.
2. The patient should be instructed to lean backward and laterally onto the image receptor.
3. The patient's arm should rest along the top of the image receptor at right angles to the body.

Position of the part:

1. The lateral aspect of the breast and the upper and outer portion of the breast should be positioned on top of the image receptor.
2. The central ray should be directed between the nipple and the axilla.
3. Compression should be applied. It may be necessary to increase exposure factors if compression is not as taut as in the craniocaudal view.

2.5. Cleavage View (CV)

The cleavage view (valley view, or medial view) is useful when examining lesions located very deep and medial to the chest wall.

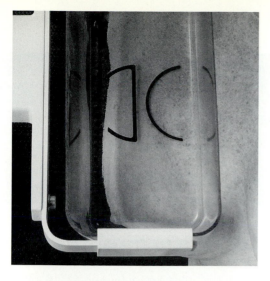

A

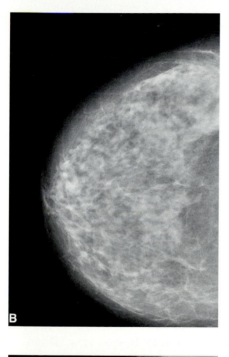

B

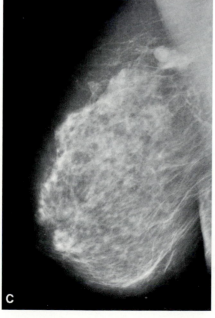

C

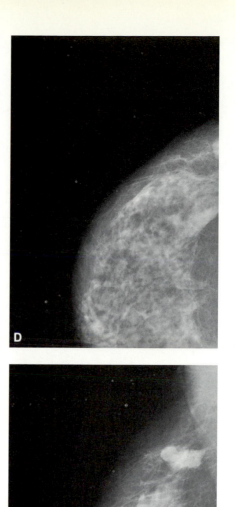

D

E

Figure 7.18. **A.** Proper positioning of the axillary tail view. After the standard craniocaudal (**B**) and mediolateral oblique views (**C**) are taken, an exaggerated craniocaudal view (**D**) and axillary tail view (**E**) are taken to further evaluate an area of suspicion in the upper outer quadrant.

Position of the patient:

1. The patient should be erect and facing the image receptor, as in the craniocaudal view.
2. The patient should be instructed to lean forward.
3. The patient's head should be turned away from the side being examined.

Procedure:

1. The image receptor should be raised to meet the inframammary crease. The breast must be perpendicular, or 90°, to the chest wall (Figure 7.19A and B).
2. Both breasts should be distributed onto the image receptor. The distribution of the breast tissue will depend upon the area of interest.
3. Compression may or may not be applied. This will depend on the location of the lesion. If compression is applied, the technologist's hand should begin to "pull" the breast tissue at the sternal notch onto the receptor.
4. The technologist may choose to mark the area of interest with a BB.

Exposure factors:

1. It may be necessary to resort to manual exposure factors. The breast tissue will not always cover the photo-cell pickup. The position of the photo cell should be checked.

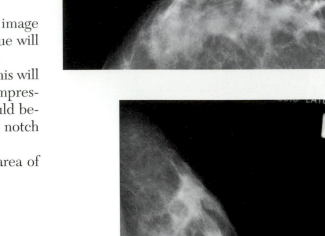

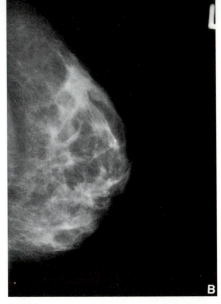

Figure 7.20. The craniocaudal view (**A**) demonstrates an area of suspicion. After taking a 90° mediolateral view (**B**), a top medial rolled craniocaudal view (**C**) and a 90° mediolateral spot magnification view (**D**) are taken to further evaluate the area in question.

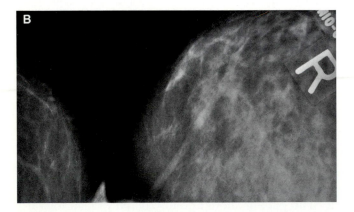

A

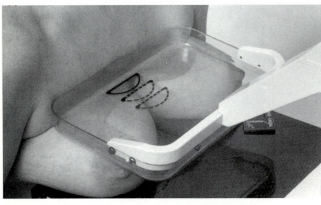

B

Figure 7.19. **A.** Proper positioning of the cleavage view. **B.** Cleavage view.

2. If the patient is not compressed, exposure factors must be increased. Manual exposure may be preferred.

2.6. Rolled (RL,RM) View

The rolled view is helpful when dense breast tissue is superimposed on a lesion (Figure 7.20A through D). The idea is to "roll" the lesion off or away from the dense tissue. Two exposures are often required. The breast is rolled in an equal and opposite direction from one view to the next (Figure 7.21A and B). In some situations it may be easier to rotate the x-ray tube assembly from plus or minus 5 to 10° instead of

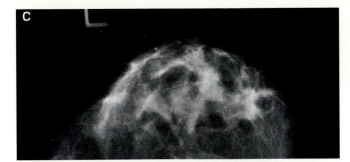

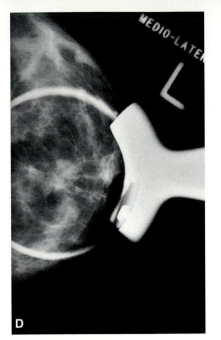

Figure 7.20.   C—D

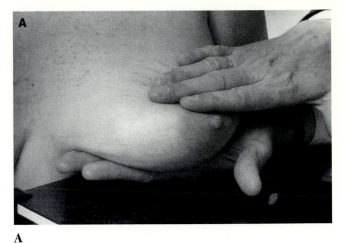

A

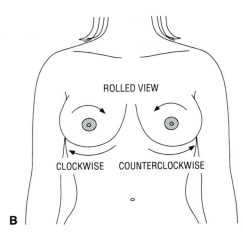

B

Figure 7.21. Various structures may be superimposed on the final image. Rolled views may assist to "roll" the area of interest off other breast tissue. **A.** Proper positioning of the rolled view. **B.** Rolled view: The patient's breasts are turned in opposite directions, about 5 to 10° in each direction.

physically manipulating the patient's breast. The rolled views may be performed in any projection. For discussion, positioning is demonstrated in the craniocaudal projection.

Position of the x-ray tube assembly:

1. The patient should be positioned as in the craniocaudal view (see Section 1.1).
2. The x-ray tube assembly should be aligned in the same fashion as in the craniocaudal view.

Procedure:

1. The patient and the breast should be positioned for the craniocaudal projection.
2. The technologist should lift the breast with one hand.
3. The other hand should be placed on top of the breast or directly opposite the first hand.

4. The technologist should rotate the breast such that her or his hands are rolling the breast in a diagonal push-pull fashion.
5. The technologist should lower the compression and begin to pull her or his hand(s) away from the breast.
6. The breast should be compressed and the exposure begun.
7. The compression should be released.
8. The exposed cassette should be removed and an unexposed cassette placed into the receptor.
9. The technologist should roll the breast in the opposite direction from the first view.
10. Compression should again be applied and the exposure taken.

(*Note:* The direction of the roll must be labeled on the film.)

2.7. Lateromedial Oblique Projection (LMO)

There are some body builds that make the standard mediolateral oblique view difficult to obtain. Patients who have a pacemaker, chest surgery, or a prominent sternum are often easier to examine in the true reverse oblique projection. A lateromedial oblique view is helpful for evaluating the medial side of the breast. The LMO view can be performed as follows.

Position of the x-ray tube assembly:

The x-ray tube assembly should be rotated from 40 to 60° for an inferior to lateral to a superior to medial projection (Figure 7.22A and B).

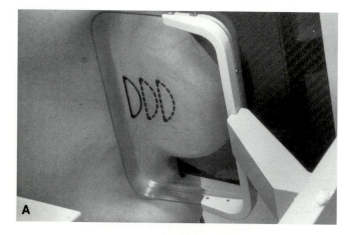

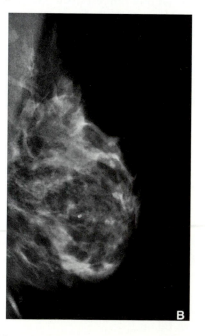

Figure 7.22. **A.** Proper positioning of the lateromedial oblique or reverse oblique view. **B.** Lateromedial oblique view.

Position of the patient:

1. The patient's sternum should be placed along the chest wall edge of the image receptor.
2. The patient's arm on the side being examined should either be raised over the top of the image receptor or placed on top of the handlebars.

Position of the part:

1. The medial aspect of the breast should be pulled up and onto the image receptor.
2. The breast should be in the lateromedial position.
3. The compression device should skim the rib cage.
4. When compression is complete, the upper outer corner of the compression device should be inferior to the humerus and at the level of the axilla.

2.8. Superolateral to Inferomedial Oblique (SIO) View

This view, formerly also called a reverse lateromedial oblique projection, is seldom utilized. If a situation warrants this view, the following will be helpful: The x-ray tube assembly should be rotated from 40 to 60° for a superior lateral to inferior medial projection (Figure 7.23). Positioning of the patient is the same as the lateromedial oblique view (see Section 2.7).

2.9. Tangential (TAN) View

The tangential view is often used to locate skin calcification or lesions that are thought to be near the skin. A BB, x-spot, or piece of lead is often placed

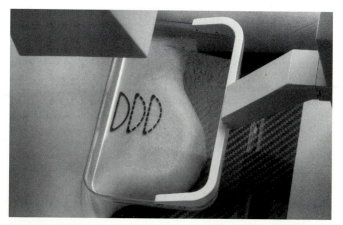

Figure 7.23. Proper positioning for the superolateral to inferomedial oblique view.

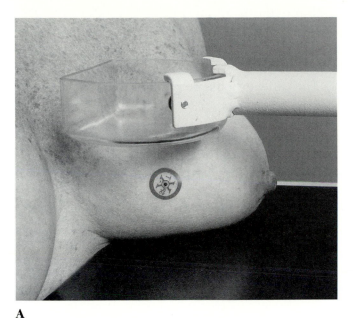

A

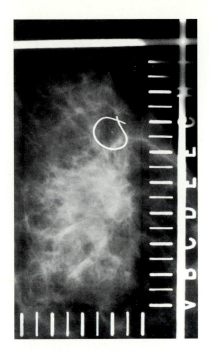

C

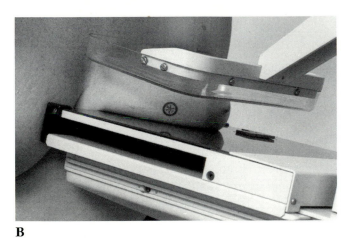

B

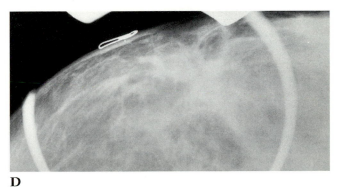

D

Figure 7.24. A tangential view may be advantageous to evaluate skin calcifications. **A** and **B.** Proper positioning for positioning of the tangential view. Utilize a spot compression device (as in **A**) or a localization compression device (as in **B**). **C.** A 90° mediolateral view taken with a localization compression paddle to determine the location of the microcalcifications in question. **D.** A tangential view of the questioned microcalcifications.

over the area of interest. If necessary, the localization grid compression paddle is used to help locate the area of interest. The central ray is directed tangential to the skin surface (Figure 7.24A through C).

Positioning of the x-ray tube assembly and the patient will depend upon where the area of interest lies. The projection should be correlated with the area of interest on the reference images. The x-ray tube assembly and the image receptor are positioned perpendicular to the area of interest. Manual exposures are often necessary, especially if the breast does not completely cover the photo cell.

2.10. Spot Compression View

The spot view (focal-spot view, coned-down spot view, or spot compression view) helps to evaluate a suspicious area. By applying focal compression and collimating the x-ray beam to the area of interest, one can improve resolution (see Figure 7.25). The spot view can be performed in any projection, including magnification. Once the routine views are evaluated and the area of interest is defined, the film projection is selected.

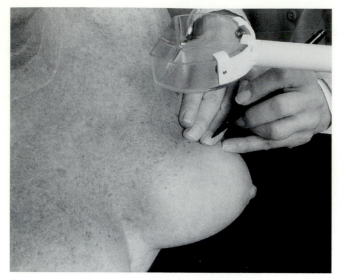

A

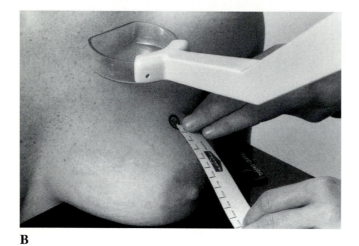

B

Figure 7.25. Spot compression. **A.** Preparing a patient with a palpable mass. **B.** Preparing the patient with a nonpalpable mass. Transfer the measurements taken from the mammogram with a tape measure.

When a spot view is taken, the compression device is changed to a smaller, often circular-shaped device. The technologist should collimate to the area of interest unless otherwise instructed by the radiologist. Sometimes it is advantageous to apply additional localized compression—for example, placing a radiolucent plastic cup lid onto the image receptor before positioning the patient. When this is done, localized compression is applied from the two sides. Double-compression spot devices are commercially available.

2.10.1. The Palpable Mass

Positioning of the part:

1. The patient should be positioned in the projection selected.
2. The area of interest can be marked with a felt-tip pen (Figure 7.25A). Or a skilled mammographer will position the patient by palpating the mass. The central ray should be directed to the area of interest.
3. Compression should be applied.

(*Note:* Remember that it may be necessary to increase exposure factors, especially when collimating to a limited area.)

2.10.2. Spot Compression View of the Nonpalpable Mass

Positioning of the part:

1. The patient should be positioned in the projection selected.
2. With a tape measure and the routine mammogram, measurements should be taken of the area of interest (Figure 7.25B).
3. The measurements taken from the mammogram should be transferred onto the patient. With a felt-tip pen, the area of interest should be marked on the patient's skin. Technologists may choose to use their fingertips as a measuring device.
4. The central ray should be directed to the marked spot on the patient's skin.

2.11. Magnification (M)

Magnification improves visibility of fine detail. It is especially useful for evaluating margins of lesions and for analyzing calcifications.

All magnification views can be done in a fashion similar to the standard projections. Patient positioning is determined as necessary to evaluate the area of interest, depending on the projection selected and the size of the area in question. The compression device selected and how much collimation will be required must be also determined. The mammographer must select the smallest focal spot and correctly

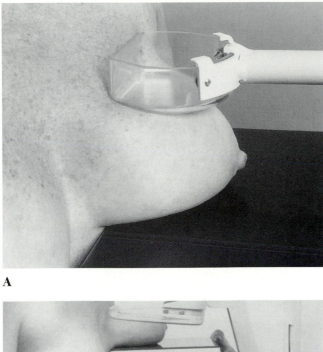

A

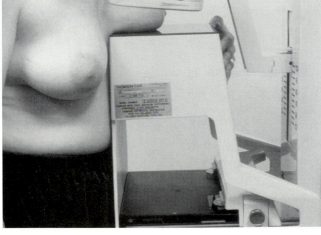

B

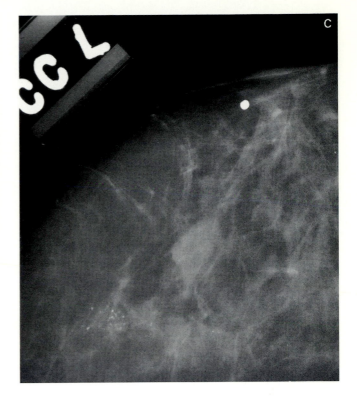

Figure 7.26. Enlarging the area of interest may improve the radiologist's ability to diagnose the patient images. **A.** Proper positioning of a magnification performed in the craniocaudal projection using spot compression. **B.** Full view magnification views may be beneficial. **C.** A magnified craniocaudal view is performed to enlarge the calcifications for further evaluation.

assemble the magnification device (Figure 7.26A through C). The exposure time is often increased compared with the routine views. The patient should hold her breath during the exposure.

2.12. Anteroposterior View

The anteroposterior view (chest wall view) has been known as the chest wall, retromammary, or axillary view. This view may be used to evaluate the chest wall, retromammary space, axilla, and deep upper structures of the breast, including the axillary nodes. This view has limited application, but some facilities take an axillary view of some patients, such as those who have had (1) mastectomies, to evaluate the surgical site, or (2) implants, to evaluate the breast tissue behind the implant (Figure 7.27A and B).

Position of the x-ray tube assembly:

1. The x-ray tube assembly should be turned from 70 to 90°.
2. The central ray should be directed from the anterior to the posterior aspect of the patient.
3. The image receptor should be raised to include the superior aspect of the head of the humerus.

Position of the patient:

1. The axilla, upper arm, posterior ribs, and breast should be positioned over the image receptor.
2. The affected arm should be abducted 90°.
3. The patient should be turned into the receptor 10 to 30°.
4. Compression may be applied and serves as a reminder to the patient to remain still.

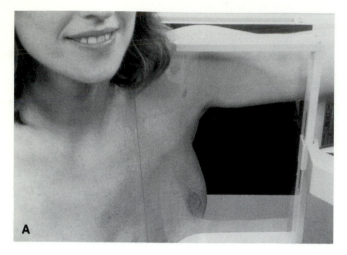

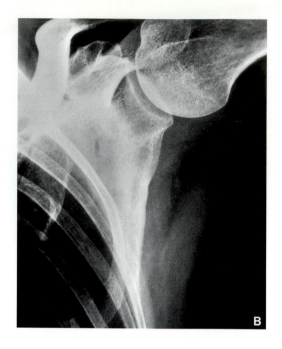

Figure 7.27. **A.** Proper positioning of the anteroposterior view. **B.** Anteroposterior view.

Exposure factors:

Adjustments in exposure factors are required to perform the axillary or the chest-wall view (Section 2.13). Depending on the equipment capabilities and the "look" the radiologist prefers, the selected kVp will range from 25 to 45. Selection of target material and/or filtration material will depend upon the equipment used (check with the equipment manufacturer for suggested exposure factors). The anteroposterior view will require exposure factors that may overpenetrate the breast tissue. A manual exposure is preferred.

>   **Example:** With Mo/Mo and Mo/Al equipment, use Mo/Al and high kVp when an image such as seen on Figure 27B is desired.

3. Mammography of the Augmented Breast

Most implants can be displaced by modified compression views (implant-displaced or ID views) to permit visualization of overlying breast tissue.

The routine for imaging the augmented breast includes:

1. The standard two views: craniocaudal and mediolateral oblique

2. The modified two views: craniocaudal and mediolateral oblique

The modified compression technique requires pulling the natural breast tissue forward (Figure 7.28A through D). Simultaneously, the implant is pushed back toward the chest wall. The technologist should remember: "pull and push." For standard views, implant included, compression is used only for immobilization. For ID views, implant excluded, compression is applied to breast tissues.

3.1. Standard Views

The standard views are first taken to demonstrate the posterior breast tissue surrounding the margins of the implant. Compression is used for immobilization only.

1. The craniocaudal view: The patient should be positioned for the routine craniocaudal view (see Section 7.1.1 for explanation). Manual exposure factors should be selected. Limited compression should be applied (Figure 7.29A and B). The anterior breast tissue will not be compressed and will be soft to the touch.

2. The mediolateral oblique view: The patient should be positioned for the mediolateral oblique view (see Section 1.2 for explanation). The appropriate manual exposure should be selected. Limited compression should be applied (Figure 7.30A and B).

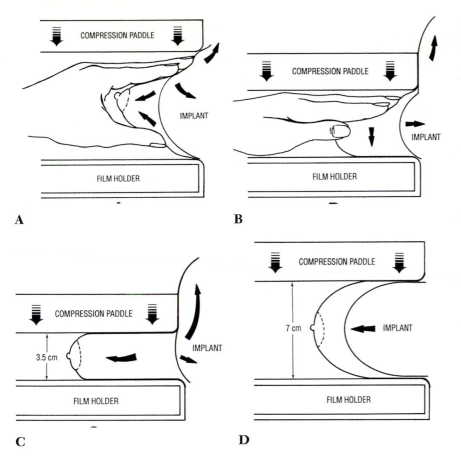

Figure 7.28. Technique and advantage of modified compression relative to limitations imposed by inclusion of implant in compression field. **A** and **B.** Modified compression views begin with pulling of breast tissue over and in front of the implant, while hand and compression paddle push implant posteriorly as breast tissue is compressed. **C.** Breast tissue has been brought into field with compression displacing implant posteriorly and excluding it from field. **D.** Breast compressed together with implant results in implant being driven forward, compacting breast tissue and significantly limiting degree of compression. Reprinted from Bushy RC, Eklund GW, Job JS, Miller SH. Improved imaging of the augmented breast. AJR 1988;151:469–473, with permission.

3.2. Modified Views

The modified views require the technologist to manipulate the breast tissue forward and push the implant back toward the chest wall to visualize additional breast tissue (Figure 7.31A).

1. The modified craniocaudal view: The patient should be positioned for the craniocaudal view. The mammographer should manipulate the breast

tissue forward (Figure 7.31A). Compression should be applied. Care must be taken so that the implant does not slide forward. The chest-wall edge of the compression device should skim the implant (Figure 7.31B and C). The AEC can be used by positioning the photo cell under the patient's breast tissue.

2. The modified mediolateral oblique view: The patient should be positioned for the MLO view. The breast tissue should be manipulated forward,

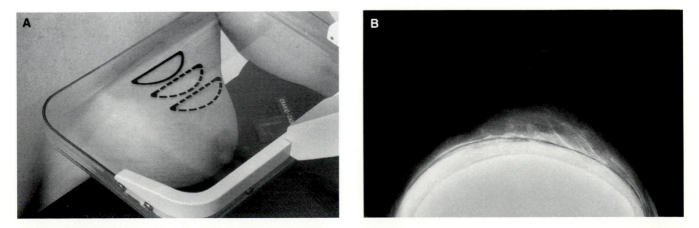

Figure 7.29. **A.** Proper positioning of a routine craniocaudal view of implant patient with minimal compression. **B.** Routine craniocaudal view—implant patient.

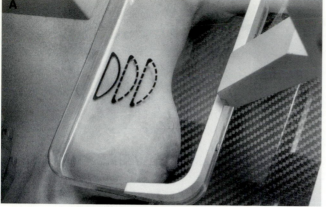

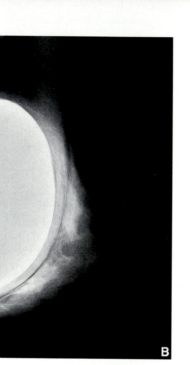

Figure 7.30. **A.** Proper positioning of the mediolateral oblique view of implant patient with minimal compression. **B.** Mediolateral oblique view—implant patient.

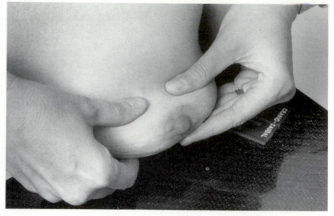

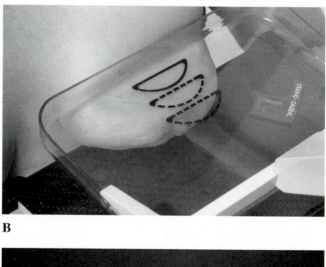

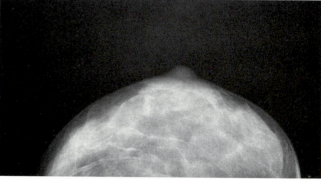

Figure 7.31. **A.** Technologist pushing implant back to the chest wall and pulling the breast tissue forward. **B.** Proper positioning of the modified craniocaudal view—Eklund technique—with compression of breast tissue. **C.** Modified craniocaudal view—Eklund technique.

pushing the implant back to the chest wall (Figure 7.32A). Compression should be applied. The compression device will slide along the border of the implant (Figure 7.32B and C). The AEC can be used as discussed above.

As in any positioning performed, the examination must be tailored to the patient. If a mediolateral view is required, the same principles for modified positioning are applied (Figure 7.33). Factors that will affect the technologist's ability to position the patient are (4):

1. The degree of encapsulation (an encapsulated implant is difficult to compress because of the scar tissue or hardening along the chest wall)
2. The size of the breast
3. The amount of natural breast tissue

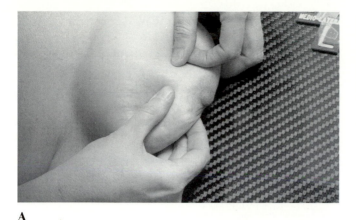

A

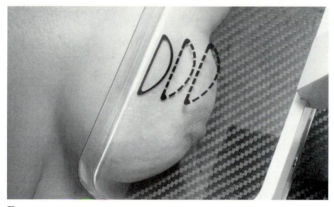

B

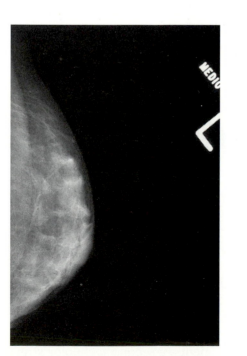

C

Figure 7.32. **A.** Technologist manipulating breast tissue forward for the mediolateral oblique view. **B.** Proper positioning of the modified mediolateral oblique view—Eklund technique. **C.** Modified mediolateral oblique view—Eklund technique.

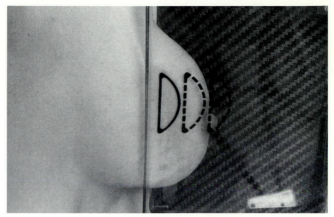

Figure 7.33. Proper positioning of the modified 90° mediolateral view— Eklund technique.

Those patients who have subpectoral or intramammory implants should be positioned in the manner discussed above. Patients with subpectoral implants may experience some discomfort during the conventional views. The patient who has a fibrous encapsulated implant may be more difficult, and the implant may restrict the amount of breast tissue that can be pulled forward. Consequently, superior and inferior tissue will be missed. A 90° lateral projection is added to the routine if the patient has this type of implant. Spot-compression views or magnification views can also be taken on implant patients.

4. Stretcher Patients

Positioning a stretcher patient is a challenge. Positioning often requires skill, imagination, and patience on the part of the technologist. Before positioning the patient, the technologist should explain to the patient what she should expect.

4.1. Craniocaudal View

1. The patient is recumbent on the stretcher and is turned on the side opposite to that which is being examined (see Chapter 8, Figure 8.4A).
2. The x-ray tube assembly is rotated 90°.
3. The inferior surface of the breast is positioned onto the image receptor. The positioning is similar to that of the craniocaudal view. The technologist must hold the breast in place. Compression is applied.

4.2. Caudocranial View

1. The patient is recumbent on the stretcher and is turned on the side opposite to that which is being examined (Figure 7.34).
2. The x-ray tube assembly is rotated 90°.
3. The superior surface of the breast is positioned onto the image receptor. The positioning is similar to that of the caudocranial view. The technologist must hold the breast in place. Compression is applied.

4.3. 90° Lateral(s)

Positioning the 90° lateral(s) will be more comfortable for the patient and may be more achievable than the oblique (see Chapter 8, Figure 8.4B).

4.3.1. Mediolateral View

1. The x-ray tube assembly is positioned at the 0° angle. The image receptor is placed on the stretcher.
2. The patient is recumbent and lying on the side to be examined. The patient's breast is carefully positioned on to the image receptor. Compression is applied.

4.3.2. Lateromedial View

1. The x-ray tube is positioned at the 0° angle.
2. The patient is recumbent and lying on the opposite side of the breast that will be examined.
3. The height of the image receptor is such that the patient's sternum is tightly against the lateral aspect of the image receptor.
4. The patient's breast is pulled over on top of the image receptor. Compression is applied.

4.4. Mediolateral Oblique View

1. If the patient is capable of sitting, the back of the stretcher is raised to support her.
2. The x-ray tube assembly is positioned parallel with the patient's pectoral muscle. The image receptor is positioned between the back of the stretcher and the patient. The patient's humerus rests on top of the image receptor. The breast is positioned on the image receptor. Compression is applied. Often, the positioning is similar to that of the axillary tail view.

Positioning a stretcher patient is often less than optimal. Thus the radiographs are not as "pretty" as those of a patient who is cooperative and can move on her own.

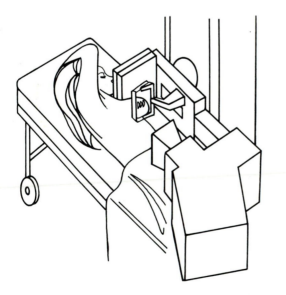

Figure 7.34. Stretcher patient having a caudocranial view performed.

5. Problems in Positioning

Not every patient is built the same way. It may become necessary to modify the normal mammography procedure to obtain all the required information. It is also important to remember that a patient who is anxious, tense, or uncooperative requires all the patience and understanding a technologist has in order to relax. In these types of situations, additional time is required for the examination.

If a patient is physically impaired—for example, a stroke patient—a second technologist may have to assist. It is helpful to establish guidelines for radiographing the difficult patient. This will alleviate unnecessary exposure and anxiety for both the patient and the technologist.

5.1. Craniocaudal Projection

5.1.1. Nipple Not in Profile

Some patients' habitus makes it difficult to position the breast with the nipple in profile. Care must be taken to make sure the image receptor is not too high or too low so the patient's breast is properly positioned. Sometimes the incorrect height of the image receptor is the reason why the nipple is not in position (Figure 7.35A through C).

If the nipple is not in profile in an otherwise properly positioned image of the full breast, the nipple should be imaged separately. One may consider the following:

1. The patient should be positioned in the craniocaudal projection. The posterior breast tissue should be pulled into position, maximizing the amount of breast to be evaluated. If desired, a nipple marker should be placed over the nipple. If this is done, the radiologist will recognize the marker and not misinterpret the nipple as a soft-tissue mass. When necessary, supplementary nipple views are taken with the nipple in profile. or
2. The breast should be positioned in the craniocaudal projection with the nipple in profile. The breast is centered to the image receptor. An additional view for the posterior breast tissue will be necessary.

Note that in Figure 7.36A the nipple is in profile. In Figure 7.36B the nipple is turned under, and in Figure 7.36C the nipple is turned up on top of the breast. Proper positioning of the full breast is preferred.

5.1.2. Skin Folds or Wrinkling of the Breast (Figure 7.37)

Skin folds under the compression paddle can be handled one of two ways:

1. The breast should be compressed. The skin folds should be gently smoothed out with the technologist's index finger. It is imperative that the posterior breast tissue not be pulled away. Present imaging techniques make the skin folds easier to penetrate and evaluate. If the area surrounding

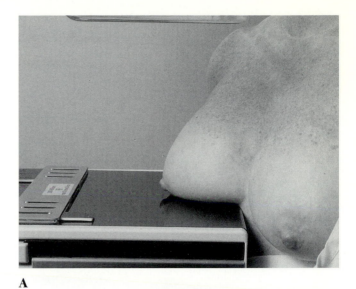

A

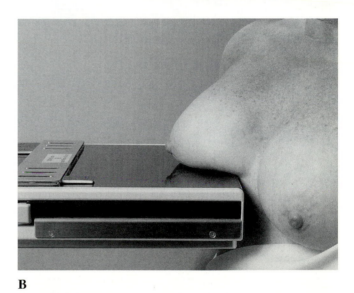

B

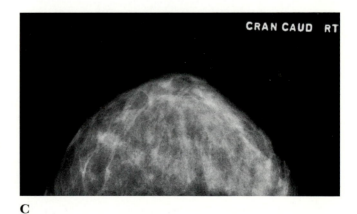

C

Figure 7.35. **A.** Craniocaudal view positioned with the receptor too low for the patient. **B.** Craniocaudal view positioned with the receptor too high for the patient. **C.** Craniocaudal view improperly positioned and the image does not demonstrate sufficient posterior breast tissue.

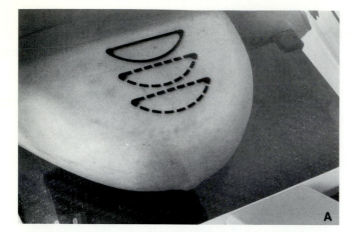

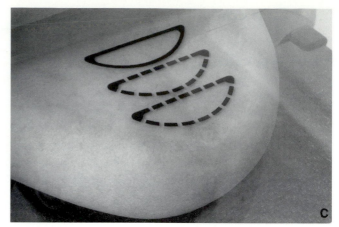

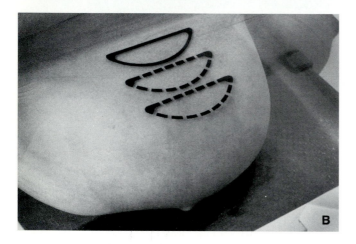

Figure 7.36. **A.** Nipple in profile. **B.** Nipple rolled on the underside of the breast. **C.** Nipple turned on top of the breast.

The arm should be relaxed following compression.
• Reposition the arm: the patient should hold onto the handlebar or should place her palm up under the image receptor.

5.1.4. Patients Difficult to Compress Due to Body Habitus

Patients who are difficult to compress for the craniocaudal view include:

• A male patient
• A young athletic female patient
• A kyphotic patient
• A patient with a pacemaker

the skin fold is suspicious, another projection may be required.
2. If the first alternative is not acceptable, the breast tissue must be smoothed out before compression is applied. Unfortunately, often breast tissue is compromised. When necessary, additional views should be taken to supplement the breast tissue eliminated from the original radiograph.

5.1.3. Lateral Skin Folds

If a patient has adipose tissue that rolls over the top of the compression paddle (Figure 7.37), the following methods to eliminate superimposition should be tried:

1. Tape the "fat roll" out of position.
2. Reposition the shoulder area of the side being examined by doing the following:
   • The patient should stand in a military position—shoulder back.
   • The arm should be abducted at right angles to the chest wall. Compression should be applied.

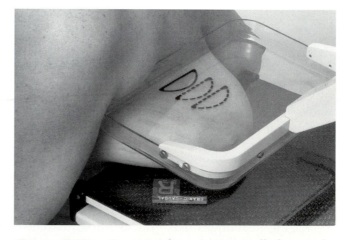

Figure 7.37. Posterior breast tissue rolled over the compression device.

The technologist should consider trying the following to improve her or his ability to compress the patient's breast:

1. If the mammography equipment is designed to do so, rotate the x-ray tube assembly 180° and perform a caudocranial projection.

   or

2. The patient should be positioned for the craniocaudal projection. The patient should relax the side of the body being examined. This can be performed by having the patient relax her shoulder, knee, and hip. When this is done, the breast tissue appears to become easier to manipulate onto the receptor.

5.2. Mediolateral Oblique View

5.2.1. Pinching the Patient in the Axilla Area

If the patient is positioned as desired but complains of pain when compression is applied, the following should be tried:

1. Compression should be released.
2. The patient should remain in position.
3. The technologist should walk behind the patient and lift the arm or axillary area and reposition the patient's arm. Sometimes the patient's pectoral muscle and latissimus dorsi muscles are improperly positioned onto the image receptor. Only the pectoral muscle should be on the image receptor and the latissimus should be placed tightly along the lateral aspect (chest wall edge) of the image receptor.
4. Reposition the breast.
5. The height of the receptor should be checked. The receptor should be lowered when necessary. The top of the receptor should be parallel to the patient's arm when abducted 90° from the body.

Note: Often "pinching" will occur in the MLO view as a result of the incorrect angle selected for the patient or as a result of not "lifting" the breast medially before placing the breast onto the compression device.

5.2.2. Incorrect or Uneven Compression

If compression can be applied to the upper half of the breast but not the lower portion:

1. The patient's build and the positioning should be reevaluated.

2. The patient should be repositioned as described in Section 6.2.1.
3. When the patient is extremely thick in the upper forearm and upper quadrants of the breast, it may be necessary to attempt other projections. For example, an axillary tail view should be taken for the upper portion of the breast. A contact lateral should be taken for the lower portion of the breast.

When the compression can be applied to the lower half of the breast but not the upper portion of the breast:

1. The patient should be reevaluated.
2. The height of the image receptor should be checked.
3. The angle of the x-ray tube assembly should be checked. The image receptor should be parallel to the pectoral muscle.
4. The patient's arm and upper breast tissue should be repositioned onto the image receptor.
5. When necessary, the standard positioning should be substituted to obtain the required information.

5.2.3. Thin Patient

A thin patient can be difficult to position for the MLO view. In such a case, the patient should be assessed. A reverse oblique view should be tried. Note the patient in Figure 7.38A and B. In the LMO view, much more of the patient's breast is visualized. It may be necessary to obtain a MLO (90° lateral) view.

Alternatives are to try the following:

1. The patient should place her arm along the top of the image receptor. If necessary, the patient's elbow should be placed behind the image receptor. This may help to bring the pectoral muscle onto the image receptor.
2. Once the patient is positioned, the height of the image receptor should be checked. The axillary region should slowly be repositioned. The posterior axillary fat should be lifted behind the image receptor.
3. The angle of the image receptor should be checked. Is the receptor parallel to the pectoral muscle?

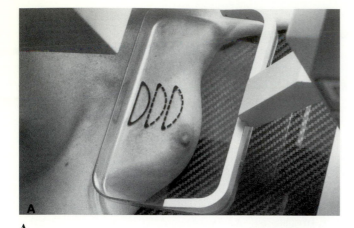

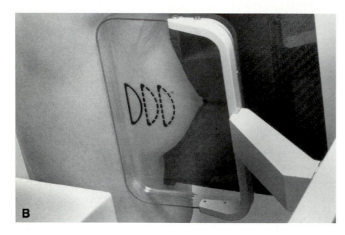

Figure 7.38. **A.** 60° mediolateral oblique view on a thin patient. **B.** Lateromedial oblique view on the same patient visualizes more breast tissue.

5.2.4. Patient with an Extremely Obese Upper Arm

To position the patient, the technologist should stand behind the patient and roll or manipulate the adipose tissue from the upper arm behind the image receptor.

5.2.5. Multiple Views Needed

When more than one view is necessary to cover the entire breast tissue:

1. The axillary tail or the MLO view should be considered for the upper half of the breast.
2. A mediolateral (90° lateral) view should be taken for the lower half of the breast.

5.2.6. Kyphotic or Pacemaker Patients

When a patient is a kyphotic or has a pacemaker:

1. A lateromedial oblique (reverse oblique) view should be considered.
   or
2. A 90° lateromedial projection should be considered for the lower half of the breast.

5.2.7. Inframammary Region Not Visualized

When the inframammary region of the breast is not visualized on the radiograph:

1. Determine if the patient's build is contributing to this or if it is due to poor positioning (Figure 7.39).
2. Have the patient stand slightly in front of the image receptor. The patient should lean back onto the receptor. The patient's hips may have been too far away from the receptor or behind the receptor.

5.2.8. Superimposition of Other Anatomy

Care must be taken not to radiograph the patient's hand, chin, nose, or the nipple from the opposite breast in the final image.

5.2.9. Incorrect Angle for the Body Part

When the angle is incorrect for the body part, the patient's build should be reevaluated. The C-arm angle should be adjusted such that the image receptor is parallel to the patient's pectoralis major. The patient should be repositioned.

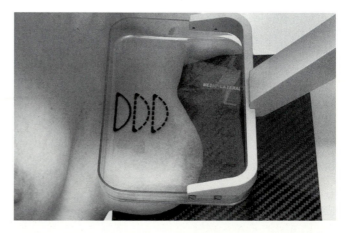

Figure 7.39. Mediolateral oblique view missing the bottom of the breast.

5.3. Mediolateral View

The most common problems seen in positioning of the mediolateral projection are as follows:

1. Image receptor too high: The height of the image receptor should be reevaluated. The patient's breast should be centered to the film. The affected arm should rest on top of the image receptor.
2. Posterior breast tissue missing: Often patients are positioned with one arm behind the image receptor. This will pull the posterior tissue away from the image receptor. The affected arm should be repositioned to rest on top of the receptor. The technologist should manipulate and position the posterior breast tissue onto the film.
3. "Drooping" breast: The patient's breast should be lifted up onto the image receptor. The breast should be held in position until compression is applied. When the breast is allowed to fall, often posterior breast tissue is missed. The final image may appear underexposed. This is usually due to improper positioning of the breast over the photocell detector.
4. Abdominal tissue not permitting proper compression and positioning of the patient: The patient should step away from the receptor slightly and should bend at the waist into the receptor or tilt the buttocks back away from the equipment.

5.4. Sectional Imaging of the Extremely Large Patient

Each facility must decide how to address those occasions when the patient is too large to allow visualization of the breast with one exposure per projection.

> **Suggestion:** The patient should be exposed by quadrants. When the various projections are sectioned, it is *essential* to label the films for proper evaluation.
>
> **Example:** mediolateral oblique projection—
> MLO upper
> MLO lower
> MLO anterior
> MLO posterior

Large patients present a challenge to the technologist. Care must be taken not to let the patient know or sense the technologist's frustration.

6. The Male Patient

The number of male patients who have mammograms is minimal. The male patient having a mammogram often has more breast tissue than a small woman. Positioning of the male patient should be handled like that of a female patient (Figure 7.40A and B).

> **Suggestion:** It may be difficult to obtain a craniocaudal view of a muscular male patient. A caudocranial view should be taken (see Section 2.1).

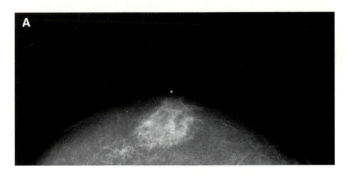

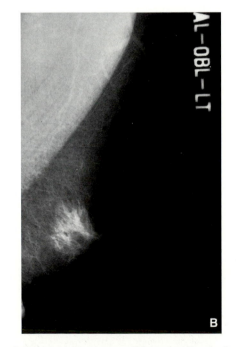

Figure 7.40. **A.** Craniocaudal view of a male patient. **B.** Mediolateral oblique view of a male patient. With proper positioning, maximal breast tissue can be visualized.

A male patient is often very embarrassed, as a mammogram is thought to be a "woman's procedure." The technologist must be sensitive to those feelings, making the patient as comfortable as possible.

7. Summary

In this chapter, positioning has been discussed. It is imperative that the mammographer assess the patient and tailor the examination to the patient. When a facility begins to perform mammography, it must decide on the standard views to be implemented. If a patient requires supplemental views, the technologist must determine how the patient will be handled to take extra projections.

References

1. Andersson I. Medical Radiology and Photography. Rochester, NY: Eastman Kodak; 1986;62:10–18.
2. Feig SA. The importance of supplementary mammographic views to diagnostic accuracy. AJR 1988;151:40–41.
3. Sickles EA. Practical solutions to common mammographic problems: Tailoring the examination. AJR 1988;151:31–39.
4. Bushy RC, Eklund GW, Job JS, Miller SH. Improved imaging of the augmented breast. AJR 1988; 151:469–473.

8

Special Procedures in Mammography

With the increase in the number of screening procedures, the number of special procedures in mammography has increased. Lesions are often diagnosed early enough to allow breast conservation therapy. The procedures discussed in this chapter are as follows:

- ultrasound
- ductography
- cyst aspiration
- pneumocystography
- preoperative wire localization
- fine needle aspiration
- stereotactic needle localization
- specimen radiography

1. Teamwork

The procedures listed above require teamwork and organization. The team consists of the radiologist, surgeon, pathologist, cytologist, and technologist. Some of the procedures, such as specimen radiography, will require cooperation between the operating room (OR) and the radiology department.

Communication is a "must" for these procedures to operate smoothly. Before a procedure is begun, protocols should be established by the radiologist in cooperation with the other physicians involved. The radiologist should also determine a protocol for these procedures within the mammography department.

The protocols should then be communicated to all involved.

> **Suggestion:** Each procedure should have a written protocol listing all necessary supplies and the radiographs that are usually performed during the procedure.

2. Preparation of the Patient

Before beginning a special procedure, the technologist and the radiologist should explain to the patient what to expect during the examination. Patient cooperation is extremely important during such procedures. The technologist's attitude and sensitivity are more critical during a special procedure than during the routine mammogram. For example, a patient who has a needle localization may be going to go to the OR following the visit to the mammography department. The patient is often anxious or scared. Therefore it is important that the patient be allowed to feel she is a part of the examination. She should be allowed to express her feelings, those of discomfort or anxiety. Open communication is required not only between the technologist and the patient but also between the radiologist and the patient.

3. Views Taken during Special Procedures

The original mammogram should be reviewed with the radiologist performing the special procedure. If the patient has had several mammograms, the examination that was used to determine the need for the special procedure should be reviewed. The views taken during a special procedure are directed by the radiologist performing the procedure. Normally the requested views are the craniocaudal view (Figure 8.1A and B) and a 90° lateral view (see Figure 8.4B). *Note:* Be advised, when employing adjunctive modalities such as ultrasound or nuclear medicine, that the conventional mammographic positioning is not utilized.

4. Ultrasound

Ultrasound is not used for breast cancer screening but plays an important roll as an adjunct to x-ray mammography.

The primary indication for ultrasound is to provide a more specific diagnosis; for example, to determine if a mass is a solid or a fluid-filled cyst. Breast ultrasound is heavily used for performing needle-guided procedures including excisional biopsy, cyst aspiration, and core-needle biopsy.

Whole-breast ultrasound may be helpful to determine if a patient who has implants has a leak or as an adjunctive procedure when the patient presents with radiographically dense breast tissue.

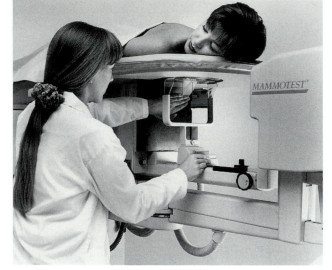

A

B

Figure 8.1. Special procedure. **A.** Craniocaudal view performed erect. Reprint courtesy of Philips Medical Systems, Shelton, CT. **B.** Craniocaudal view performed prone. Reprint courtesy of Fischer Imaging Corporation, Denver, CO.

5. Ductography

Ductography is conducted on those patients who have abnormal nipple discharge. The original mammogram should be reviewed. Scout films should be taken according to the direction of the radiologist. Usually the craniocaudal view and a 90° lateral (either mediolateral or lateromedial) view are taken (Figure 8.2A and B).

The lactiferous duct from which the discharge exudes is carefully cannulated. A small amount of contrast medium is injected into the duct. Radiographs are taken once the dye has been injected. Normally, the requested views will be a craniocaudal and a 90° lateral projection. Sometimes these views will be performed with magnification.

The purpose of a ductogram is not to determine if a lesion is benign or malignant but to determine the location(s) and number of lesions.

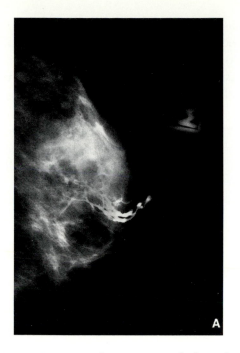

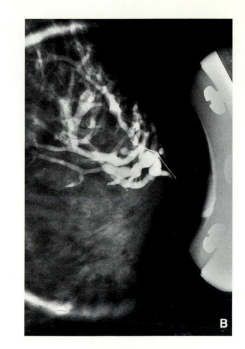

Figure 8.2. Ductography. **A.** 90° mediolateral view. **B.** Magnified mediolateral view.

6. Cyst Aspiration/ Pneumocystography

Many women develop cysts in their breasts. Sometimes it is necessary to evaluate the cyst for debris or abnormal growth. After the routine mammogram is reviewed, scout films taken with the biopsy paddle may be helpful in accurately locating the cyst in question.

The cyst is aspirated or emptied by performing a needle aspiration. Air is then injected to evaluate the inner wall of the cyst. The wall of the cyst may be smooth, or an abnormal mass may be present. The breast tissue surrounding the cyst is also evaluated. Images will be taken at the direction of the radiologist. *Note:* Facilities may choose to perform cyst aspirations under ultrasound.

7. Fine Needle Aspiration (FNA)

With the increased concern over the number of biopsies performed, attempts are being made to reduce the number of surgical procedures. Fine needle aspiration (FNA) is performed to obtain cellular material from the area in question for cytologic analysis. The accuracy of FNA is dependent on the individual performing the procedure: the radiologist, cytologist, or surgeon. Usually the technologist will be requested to take scout films of the suspicious area. Several series of films may be taken during the procedure. The views usually taken will be the craniocaudal and a 90° lateral projection with or without magnification (see Chapter 7, Section 2.11) *Note:* Often this procedure is performed with ultrasound guidance.

8. Preoperative Wire Localizations

Preoperative needle localizations are usually performed on nonpalpable abnormalities such as occult lesions or suspicious microcalcifications. The surgeon usually cannot "feel" the lesion. The needle localization allows him or her to localize an area with minimal removal of breast tissue. The needle localization is carried out by the radiologist assisted by a technologist.

The routine mammogram should be reviewed

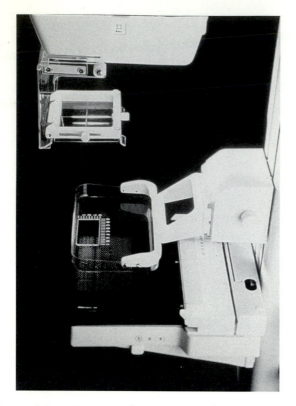

Figure 8.3. Biopsy grid compression device and biopsy light localizer. Reprint courtesy of General Electric Medical Systems, Milwaukee, WI.

with the radiologist. The scout films that are to be performed are determined. Most mammography machines have biopsy grid localizers that help the radiologist position the biopsy needle. Scout films can be taken with the biopsy grid and the light localizer (Figure 8.3A and B). Usually craniocaudal and 90° lateral views are taken. A sample procedure is described below (see Section 8.1).

Many needles are available for localizations. The choice of needle guides is determined by the radiologist and the surgeon. Examples of needle styles available on the market are the straight needle, the hookwire system, or the "anchored" needle.

The approach for performing the procedure is the decision of the radiologist.

Example: The superior-to-inferior approach done in the craniocaudal projection or the lateral-to-medial approach done in the lateromedial projection.

The patient should be seated during the needle localization unless she is placed on a biopsy table.

Images are taken during the procedure under the direction of the radiologist. A final set of films is taken to demonstrate the location of the needle in relationship to the lesion. This set of films or copies is provided for the surgeon to review during surgery.

> **Suggestion:** The sequence of films taken should be numbered with lead numbers. This will eliminate confusion when the films are sorted.

Before the patient is sent to surgery, the wire should be taped to the breast. The patient should be told to limit upper body motion. The technologist should remember to keep the patient informed of what she should expect each step of the way, from the time she enters the mammography section until she leaves.

8.1. Example of Procedure for Needle Localization

1. The area of interest and the projection(s) to be taken should be determined.
2. Scout films should be taken before each procedure.
   - As a rule, a craniocaudal and 90° lateral view must be taken (Figure 8.4A through D).
   - The localization paddle should be used in the projection in which the radiologist will begin the procedure. Spot-compression devices may be helpful for lesions located in very difficult areas.
   - The breast should be kept compressed while the scout films are checked.
   - When necessary, imaging can be done with magnification.
3. The patient should be prepared. Usually the patient is seated during the needle localization.
4. The approach for performing the procedure should be the decision of the radiologist.
5. The radiologist should place the needle.
6. Under the direction of the radiologist, a radiograph to determine needle placement should be taken. Compression should be maintained until the image is reviewed. If the radiologist is satisfied with the needle placement, the compression device should slowly and gently be removed. The patient's breast should be supported to minimize motion of the breast while the mammography equipment is repositioned for the next projection.

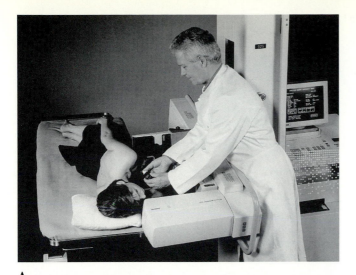

A

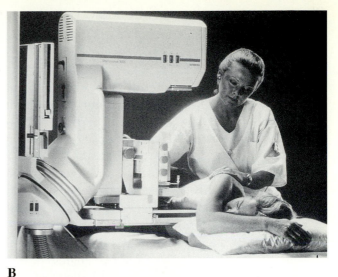

B

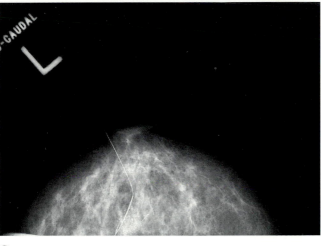

C

D

Figure 8.4. Needle localization. **A.** Stretcher patient having a craniocaudal view performed. Reprint courtesy of Philips Medical Systems, Shelton, CT. **B.** Stretcher patient having a 90° lateromedial view performed. Reprint courtesy of Siemens Medical Systems, Iselin, NJ. **C.** Craniocaudal view after needle placement. **D.** Mediolateral view after needle placement.

7. The x-ray machine should be rotated 90° from the entrance projection. The patient should be positioned. The breast should be supported and compressed slowly. This view is made to determine depth of needle penetration. The breast should remain compressed while the film is developed unless this is difficult or uncomfortable for the patient. The radiologist should review the film to determine positioning of the needle.

8. Directions for imaging should come from the radiologist until the procedure is completed. When the procedure is completed, a final set of images must be taken, marked, and sent with the patient to the OR.

9. Stereotactic Needle Localization

Several manufacturers of mammography equipment have introduced computerized localization devices. The stereotactic equipment today is available in two options:

1. A device that is an adjunctive piece of equipment mounted onto the existing mammography unit (Figure 8.5A). Once attached, it permits the patient to be compressed with a special compression device.

2. Or a facility can purchase a stereotactic prone table (Figure 8.5B). Unlike the device above, this piece of equipment is designed exclusively for image-guided tissue sampling. The stereotactic device permits the x-ray tube to be shifted to provide images of the lesion from two angles: $\pm 15°$ (stereo). These images (Figure 8.6) allow calcula-

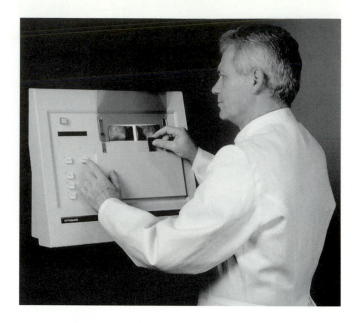

Figure 8.6. A scout film is taken at $\pm 15°$. The image(s) are placed onto the device used to calculate the coordinates for the correct placement of the needle. Reprint courtesy of Philips Medical Systems, Shelton, CT.

tion of the spatial coordinates of the lesion and determination of the position of the device guiding the biopsy needle.

Note: Today the stereo-guided equipment is capable of image acquisition by either the screen-film or digital method. Film images are acquired in the conventional manner: an x-ray of the area of interest is recorded on film. The digital method has an acquisition device (usually a charge-coupled device, or CCD) housed in the image receptor, which permits the image information to be transferred to and reviewed on a CRT monitor.

The needle is placed into the needle guide. Once the calculation has determined the proper coordinates, the needle-placement device directs and positions the needle. Those facilities with an active cytology department find the stereotactic device to be beneficial for FNA (see Section 7).

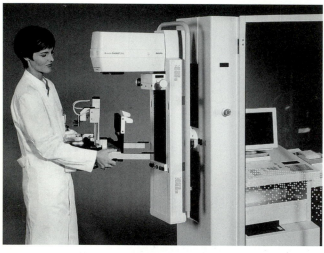

A

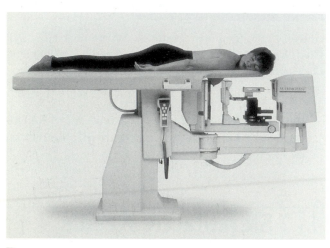

B

Figure 8.5. **A.** Stereotactic device mounted onto the Philips Diagnost 3000. Reprint courtesy of Philips Medical Systems, Shelton, CT. **B.** Prone biopsy table, Mammotest. Reprint courtesy of Fischer Imaging Corporation, Denver, CO.

10. Specimen Radiography

During a breast biopsy, a tissue sample is surgically removed and sent to the radiology department for evaluation. The radiograph confirms that the surgeon has removed the breast tissue from the area in question (Figure 8.7). The patient is usually under anesthesia; therefore speed, promptness, and efficiency are important. Each facility should establish a procedure best suited to its needs.

> **Suggestion 1:** Some facilities use a alpha-numeric grid system to establish coordinates for the pathologist.
>
> **Suggestion 2:** Compression should be applied.
>
> **Suggestion 3:** Some surgical supply companies have radiolucent containers for specimen work.

Magnification of the specimen is extremely helpful for visualizing microcalcifications. Unless the specimen is the entire breast, the grid is not necessary. Manual exposures with low kVp are preferred (see Chapter 6, "Techniques in Screen-Film Mammography").

11. Postoperative Follow-up

Follow-up mammograms are important for patient management. Each facility should establish a proto-col for how it is going to follow up the postoperative patient. For example:

1. Some facilities will include magnification views: a craniocaudal and a 90° lateral view of the surgical site on lumpectomy patients.
2. As seen in Figure 8.8A and B, a fine piece of wire can be placed over the surgical site to mark the scar. This is helpful in identifying scar tissue.
3. On postmastectomy patients, a mediolateral oblique of the remaining tissue is occasionally useful but not cost-effective as a general practice.

Every effort should be made to get to know the patient and her medical history related to her breast. When this is done, the number of additional views taken may be reduced.

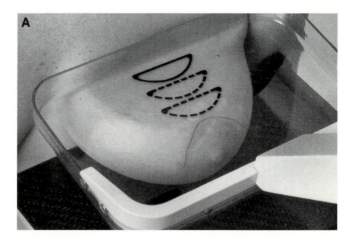

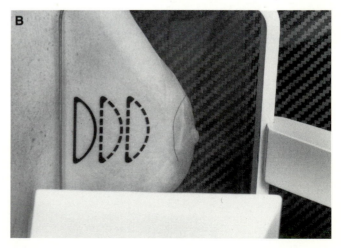

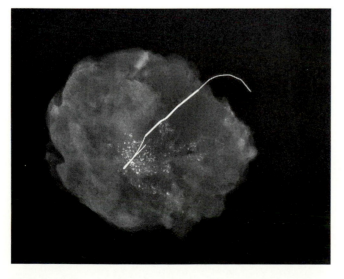

Figure 8.7. Specimen radiography of the area visualized in Figure 8.4. C and D.

Figure 8.8. **A.** Craniocaudal view of a postoperative patient. The wire marks the scar on the patient's breast. **B.** Mediolateral view with a wire marker on the surgical scar.

12. Summary

Each facility must establish the method and approach to special procedures. Protocols must be established and written up. Most of the procedures are performed by the radiologist. Decisions regarding each procedure (for example, the needle type and the images to be taken) must come from the individual performing it. Open communication is a must during a special procedure. This will permit the technologist to assist the radiologist instead of "scrambling" for what is needed. Care and precision are required to number the sequence in which the films are taken. Both the technologist and the radiologist must communicate with the patient during the procedure. The patient must cooperate during the procedure. (*Note:* For additional information, the technologist should consult with a radiologist for available literature written by key mammographers on these procedures.)

9

Quality Assurance and Quality Control

Women must be assured that they will receive mammographic examinations of the highest quality with the lowest possible risk. This goal can be achieved by implementing an extensive and comprehensive quality-assurance program. Such a program must include not only the technical testing but also peer review, image quality evaluation, and continuing education for the radiologists, technologists, and medical physicist.

In this chapter, aspects of quality assurance required to maintain the highest standard of image quality are discussed. Each facility establishing a quality-assurance program should consult the country, state, provincial or federal guidelines—for example, the Mammography Quality Standards Act (MQSA) and its appointed accrediting bodies, such as the American College of Radiology (ACR)—for specific and up-to-date information.

1. Definitions

Before a quality-assurance program is discussed, several terms must be defined.

- *Quality assurance* (QA) is the overall management of actions taken to consistently provide consistently high image quality.
- *Quality control* (QC) is the "segment of quality assurance responsible for the measurement of the image quality and the integrity of the equipment"(1).
- *Preventive maintenance* (PM) is the action taken on a regularly scheduled basis to prevent deterioration of image quality or any breakdown in the imaging chain.
- *Corrective maintenance* is the action taken to eliminate potential or actual problems.
- *Standards* are reference objects or devices with known precision used to check the accuracy of other measurement devices. These measurement devices must be calibrated against standards known to be certain, accurate, or consistent.
- *Tolerance* is the amount of measurement variation allowed under normal operating circumstances.
- *Trends* are serial measurements that follow a pattern of increase or decrease that might lead to out of limits.
- *Feedback* is the process of implementing corrective action.

2. Establishing Standards for Image Quality

Standards for image quality must be established. Image quality is subject in part to the individual reader's personal taste. However, each facility must also establish image quality standards that comply with regulatory requirements. When standards for a QA program are established, there are two levels of the evaluation:

1. The process required to monitor the performance of the imaging chain
2. A review of the effectiveness of the program itself

2.1. Available Programs

Many countries, states, or provinces have their own QA compliance programs or are currently in the process of developing similar programs. Facilities must check with their appropriate regulatory bureaus for further information.

The ACR in 1987 established a voluntary national mammography accreditation program. Because of the concern expressed over mammographic quality by both the medical community and the public, it became evident that there was a need to regulate image quality (2). The ACR program offers peer review of a facility. This program has four segments that must be completed by the site wishing to achieve accreditation:

1. A survey form must be completed by the facility. The requested information is submitted to the ACR.
2. Phantom images are submitted to evaluate image quality. The ACR at present uses the RMI 156 phantom.
3. The thermoluminescent dosimetry chip is exposed to determine radiation dose. The chip is placed on top of the RMI phantom.
4. The facility submits clinical images for evaluation by a panel of radiologists. Once the initial paperwork has been submitted and approved, a facility must submit 30 days of sensitometry or processor QC documentation. Once the account receives ACR approval, the facility is issued a 3-year certification. On an annual basis, the ACR will send the facility forms to update their site information.

In 1992, the federal government passed the MQSA to assure quality mammography on a national level. As of October 1, 1994, it was unlawful to perform mammography within the United States without first obtaining Food and Drug Administration (FDA) certification. The FDA, which was appointed as the administrative organization of the MQSA, began enforcing MQSA with an interim set of rules. The final regulations are expected to go into effect in 1996. These interim rules resulted from pressure to put a set of mammography standards into place, leading the FDA to adopt regulations closely resembling those of the ACR MAP program.

To become certified by the FDA, facilities providing mammography must be accredited by an FDA-approved accrediting body. At the time of this writing, the FDA-approved accrediting bodies are the states of California, Arkansas, Iowa, and Illinois and the ACR. The Health Care Finance Administration (HCFA), which performed on-site inspections of facilities providing screening mammography, was terminated as of October 1, 1994. Facilities providing mammography must openly display their FDA certification.

Canada is in the process of implementing its certification program. In Europe, the European Guidelines have presented a set of standards for centers of excellence. Simultaneously, individual countries are establishing regulations (i.e., France and Germany).

3. How to Institute a Quality-Assurance Program

Establishing a QA program for mammography is similar to establishing one for a large radiology facility. The Bureau of Radiological Health and other regulatory bodies have guidelines to help facilities establish the groundwork for a QA program.

First and most important, a facility must have the *commitment* from administration or upper management to support such an endeavor. This commitment requires the allocation of personnel and time to perform the required testing and funds to purchase the necessary equipment.

3.1. Initial Setup

It should be understood that the initial phase of establishing guidelines and criteria for a QA program is the most time-consuming. The success of any program depends on organization, and this also applies to quality-assurance programs.

One individual must be designated the responsible party for the entire QA and QC program. Most regulations specify that this individual should be a radiologist who has been assigned to be in charge of the QA program. This individual's responsibilities may include any or all of the following:

1. Ensure that a QA and QC program is implemented.
2. Select the person who will be the QC technologist and establish who will be performing the various QC test procedures. This includes selecting a medical physicist to direct the QC program and perform the required test procedures.
3. Provide the appropriate training and continuing education as needed by all personnel to perform their designated responsibilities. For example, for the mammography technologists, this should include (a) an orientation program encompassing departmental policy and procedures as established in the QA manual and (b) adequate training (both didactic and clinical "hands on") in mammography, meeting all regulatory requirements.
4. Establish a chain of command and file this in the QA manual.
5. Provide the test equipment required for QC testing.
6. Ensure that the appropriate time and staffing have been included in the schedule, not only to perform the QC tests but also to interpret and record the test results.
7. Provide direction to all aspects of the mammography imaging chain, including the QA and QC programs. This should include frequent feedback, both positive or negative, as appropriate. Review the QC tests on a routine basis or as needed, those performed by the QC technologists as well as those done by the medical physicist.
8. Arrange to have someone monitor the radiation protection program in conjunction with or apart from the main radiology department (this will depend on facility's size and needs).
9. Ensure that all records/documentation in the QC manual are up to date (see Section 3.2).
10. Review results regularly; ie., quarterly.
11. Provide motivation and direction.

3.2 Manual(s)

The next step in establishing a QA program is to compile the necessary documentation for the records. A policy and procedures manual or a QA/QC control manual should be developed. The manual should be written in such a way that it will be convenient to revise. The manual must be accessible to all personnel. If the decision is made to have two manuals, it may be feasible to use one manual to hold all management-related records and the second as the working QC manual. *Note:* See Figure 9.1 for one of the commercially available policy and procedure manuals.

The QA manual must contain the following information:

1. A copy of the regulations to which you are to adhere or a statement of where these regulations can be found.
2. A list of all individuals responsible for testing, supervising, repairing, or servicing the equipment. Establish who will maintain the mammography equipment—for example, the processor. Will maintenance be provided by a local processor service company or in-house personnel? Include in this section a log of telephone numbers and how to contact the involved parties.

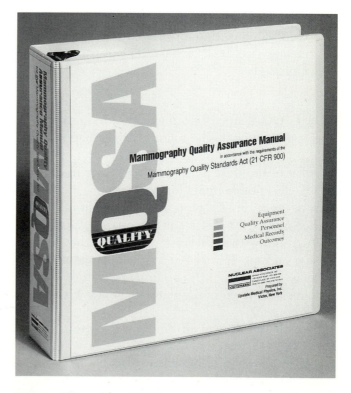

Figure 9.1. The MQSA manual. Courtesy of Nuclear Associates, Carle Place, NY.

3. A list of all individuals involved in the mammography team: the radiologists, the technologists, and the medical physicist(s). This should include employee qualifications and other information as required by the regulatory agency.
4. A list of all equipment used for mammography procedures (dedicated mammography equipment, processors, etc.) as well as all the equipment used for testing of that mammography equipment.
5. Installation records, including the initial acceptance tests (e.g., Bureau of Radiological Health testing acceptance testing).
6. Records showing maintenance of test equipment. All test equipment used during a QC program requires maintenance. Recommendations for recalibration must be followed. All repairs must also be documented.
7. A list of available reference material, including where it is located. For example, the mammography equipment service manual.
8. Radiation safety policy and procedures.
9. Documentation of committee meetings and continuing education training.
   - Committee meetings are a method of communication. All aspects of the QA program should be reviewed. As necessary, revision must be made.
   - Training is a requirement for the entire mammography team. Document all training conducted within the department as well as classes, lectures, or any educational programs attended.

The QC manual becomes the working manual, thus it must include the following information:

1. A list of the tests performed and their frequency.
2. The acceptable limits for each test.
3. A description of each test and procedure.
4. Records of the test results. Most regulatory bodies require that the test results for the current year be kept. It is a good idea to document a summary of each year the equipment is in operation. Check with your regulatory agency for its requirements.
5. Documentation of difficulties detected during testing.
6. Documentation of the corrective actions taken to resolve problems.
7. Documentation of the effectiveness of the corrective actions taken.

4. Required Components of Quality Assurance

Several components must be monitored to attain and maintain a high level of image quality. The factors that influence image quality are (3):

1. The performance of the dedicated mammography unit
2. The darkroom
3. The recording system (cassettes, film, and screens)
4. The performance of the processing systems (processor, chemistry)
5. Image analysis
   - Phantom images
   - Retake analysis
   - Continuous assessment of image adequacy
6. The view box and viewing conditions
7. Stock rotation and storage conditions
8. Personnel
   - Mammography radiologic technologist(s)
   - Radiologist(s)
   - Medical physicist(s)

The *parameters* to be monitored are as follows:

Mammography equipment:

1. Mammography unit
2. Beam quality: Half-value layer (HVL)
3. Accuracy and reproducibility of kVp
4. Accuracy and reproducibility of timer
5. Linearity and reproducibility of mA station
6. Reproducibility of x-ray tube or radiation (R) output
7. Accuracy of source-to-image distance (SID) and compression indicators
8. Collimation
9. Focal spot size
10. Compression
11. AEC performance and reproducibility
12. Grid(s)

The darkroom:

1. Darkroom integrity
   - Cleanliness
   - Airflow, ventilation, room temperature, and humidity

2. Darkroom fog
   - Safelight filter
   - Light leaks
3. Film storage bin(s)
   - Cleanliness
   - Light leaks

The recording system:

1. Cassette/Screen
   - Identification
   - Cleaning
   - Light leaks
2. Film
   - Storage and working conditions, including storage of films after development
   - Handling
3. Screen
   - Condition
   - Speed uniformity
   - Screen-film contact

Performance of the processing system:

1. Daily Processor QC
   - Mid-density or speed index
   - Density difference or contrast index
   - Base plus fog
   - Solutions' temperature(s)
   - Replenishment rates
2. Analysis of fixer retention in film
3. Processor maintenance
   - Routine maintenance
   - Daylight systems
4. Chemistry

The viewing conditions:

1. View boxes
   - Cleanliness
   - Uniformity
   - Luminance and color temperature
2. Viewing room
   - Ambient light–illuminance
   - Masking

The entire system

1. Dose calculations
2. Phantom imaging
3. Retake analysis
4. Artifact analysis

The personnel:

1. The radiologic technologist(s) performing mammography must
   - Be certified by the American Registry of Radiologic Technologists (ARRT) or have passed the appropriate regulatory accreditation licensure.
   - Have had specific training in mammography as defined by the regulatory body.
   - Maintain continuing education in mammography as defined by the regulatory body.
   - Routinely perform mammography to maintain level of competence. It has been suggested that a minimum of 20 mammograms per week be performed.
2. The Radiologist(s) must
   - Be board-certified.
   - Meet the required training to read mammograms per the regulatory description.
   - Maintain continuing education as defined by the regulatory body.
   - Routinely read a minimum of 40 mammograms per month.
3. The medical physicist must
   - Be a board-certified medical physicist or have met the qualifying requirements of the regulatory body.
   - Meet the regulatory requirements to perform a facility's physics evaluations.
   - Maintain continuing education as defined by the regulatory body.

5. Tips Before Beginning a Quality Control Program

Before beginning the actual QC testing, there are a number of tips that will help to make the procedures run more smoothly.

5.1. Frequency of the Test Procedures

Upon reviewing the regulations and their QC test procedures, normally a frequency to perform these tests will be noted. Be advised that this is the least or minimum number of times the tests should be performed.

For an individual in the learning phase of doing the test procedures, there is a learning curve. The more often the test is performed, the more competence increases. At the same time, the individual doing the QC test has the opportunity to accumulate additional data that may give indications of patterns that may be seen.

For example, if the phantom image is to be performed on a monthly basis, initially one may try doing the test once a week. A test procedure that may take 15 min in the beginning may take 5 min within a few weeks. Simultaneously the QC technologist can assess the entire imaging system's quality more often, looking for changes that may be occurring in the imaging chain. With experience, the time needed to evaluate the phantom image will decrease.

5.2. Allocation of Time to Perform the Test Procedures

At the beginning of each new QC year, mark on the calendar the dates on which all the tests should be performed. This acts as a reminder to all involved but also permits immediate scheduling of the appropriate times. For example, the annual evaluation may take 6 h. Mark off this time in the patient-schedule log book.

Those test procedures that are to be performed routinely/daily are to be done before any patient films are taken but after the appropriate warm-up has been completed. Turn all equipment on upon opening up or entering the department.

5.3. Darkroom Maintenance

The darkroom can be the cause of many unwanted problems in mammography. Often the darkroom becomes the storage area for the department; also, the design of the darkroom often creates additional problems.

The darkroom is designed for the handling of film before and after exposure as well as before and after development. The following are important points to be considered:

5.3.1. Cleanliness

Mammography images are very sensitive to artifacts. Maintenance of cleanliness should include not only the countertop where the cassettes are loaded and unloaded but also the tops of the safelight and room

lights, where dust can collect. Chemicals can be spilled or may leak, leaving a dry chemical dust. Storage bins above the counter can attract dust and dirt that is pulled down onto the counter. Film bins should be cleaned on a routine basis. The exhaust fans and vents should be kept clean. Eating and smoking must not be permitted in the darkroom.

How to maintain darkroom cleanliness is discussed in Section 7.1.

5.3.2. Construction of the Darkroom

Air conditioning and heat vents should not be installed over the workbench or the processor feed tray.

The ceiling should be made of a solid material such as plastered drywall. Ceiling tiles will create dust and may fall on the surfaces below, especially if the tiles have not been well anchored in their metal frame. Depending upon the type of door used and how it opens, often, when it is closing or opening, an air vacuum causes the tiles to lift, shaking the dust free.

It is best to store film and chemicals in a separate area outside of the darkroom. Storage areas should not be installed over the counter. If they are already there, doors should be installed to minimize the amount of dirt that might fall from the shelves to the countertops. The cardboard boxes that chemicals and film are often shipped in create additional dust into the atmosphere of the darkroom. If storage areas are available, clean them routinely.

Pass boxes, which are also dust traps, must be cleaned routinely.

Air cleaners/purifiers can assist in reducing dirt/dust in the darkroom. Static discharge systems are also available if needed. The darkroom must be kept at a given temperature and humidity year around. See section.

Ensure that the darkroom has the correct ventilation, both in and out.

5.4. Film and Chemistry Storage

5.4.1. Storage of Preexposed Film (Figure 9.2)

Film is sensitive to aging and external radiation. The film must be kept away from the radiation field. It should be kept in a dark, cool area. Make a note of the expiration date on the film boxes. This is especially important if there is a holding facility for film outside the department. Inform the stockroom that

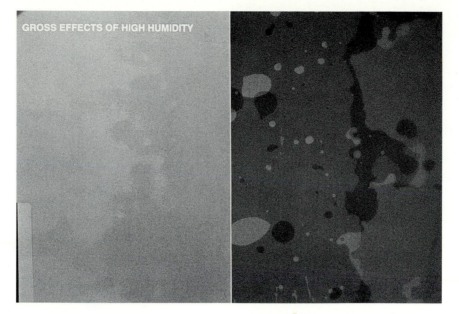

GROSS EFFECTS OF HIGH HUMIDITY

Figure 9.2. Improper storage conditions after a box of mammography film has been opened, showing the effects of high humidity and temperature in the darkroom. **A.** The visual effect on the unexposed film. **B.** After exposure, the effect of the humidity may resemble a processor-related problem.

it is important to rotate the stock. When new stock is brought into the department, it must not be used first. The old stock should be used before the new: first in, first out. If the stock is outdated, it should be discarded.

Film storage recommendations are as follows:

- *Temperature:* Less than 24°C (75°F); preferably between 15 and 21°C (60 to 70°F).
- *Humidity:* Open boxes should be stored at between 40 to 60%. See Figure 9.2.
- *Environment:* Should not be exposed to radiation or chemical fumes.
- *Storage:* Film must be stored on end to avoid pressure damage. Film should be stored by emulsion number and expiration date.

5.4.2. Storage of Postexposure Film

The archival quality of film is dependent not only on the processing conditions but also on the storage conditions after processing. The storage condition for film after processing, routinely not discussed in medical imaging, is important so as to ensure that the film has a useful archival period (a minimum of 10 years).

- *Temperature:* The best temperature for film storage film is 20°C (68°F). Film should not be stored above 25°C (77°F) for extended periods. Storage

temperatures above ± 38°C may permanently reduce the pliability of film bases. If the temperature drops below 0°C (32°F) the film will become brittle.
- *Humidity:* Humidity levels above 60% can damage the gelatin emulsion layer as a result of the growth of fungus and eventually cause the sticking of the emulsion. Exposure to high humidity will also accelerate any effects of residual processing chemistry. Conversely, consistent exposure to low humidities below 15% tends to produce temporary brittleness in the gelatin emulsion as well as an increase in potential for adhesion defects. The best condition for film storage is a relative humidity between 30 and 60%.
- *Environmental conditions:* It is essential to have good housekeeping, minimizing dust and dirt. The walls should be designed to prevent the accumulation of moisture on the interior surfaces. Facilities with air conditioning should have automatic systems. Filters should be cleaned on a routine basis.

5.4.3. Storage and Rotation of Chemistry

Facilities that purchase chemistry in concentrate, delivered in a cardboard case with several parts; such as Part A, B, and C, *must* ensure that the batches within a case are kept together in storage and when mixing the solutions. Too often, when the chemistry is delivered, someone within the department removes the contents and places it into a storage area. Chemistry *must* be mixed in the delivered unit batch. Intermixing of the chemistry batches has been known to be a source of problems with sensitometry when performing processor quality control (PQC).

5.5. Film Handling

It is recommended that, when handling films that are stored, the following precautions be followed:

1. Ensure that all surfaces that the film comes in contact with are clean. Dust and dirt may interfere with legibility and produce scratches.
2. When handling the film, wear white cotton gloves. This reduces the oil residual that may be left on the film.

5.6. Cassette-Screen Identification

Upon installing cassettes and screens in any department, the inside and outside of the cassette must be labeled (Figure 9.3). When labeling the screen, label it in an area where the x-ray field will permit it to be visualized, as near the ID window of the cassette. *Note:* Screen labels may cause localized defects in film-screen contact; place the labels at the periphery.

Place the same number labeled on the screen on the outside of the cassette. Most manufacturers of cassettes have a label on the back of the cassette. Label not only the cassette-screen ID number but the date the cassette was placed into operation.

The purpose of identifying the cassette-screens is to help the technologist(s) and/or radiologist(s) quickly determine which cassette-screen may be causing a problem and to remove it from operation until the problem is corrected.

5.7. Selecting the Film, Chemistry, Processor and Cycle Time for Development

Each company has developed its product to best operate in "its" conditions. A number of companies develop these products. Before using the products for patients, confer with the manufacturer to determine the appropriate processing "system" to obtain the best results.

When it is necessary to combine products from several companies, the facility must understand that they may be compromising quality (see Chapter 4,

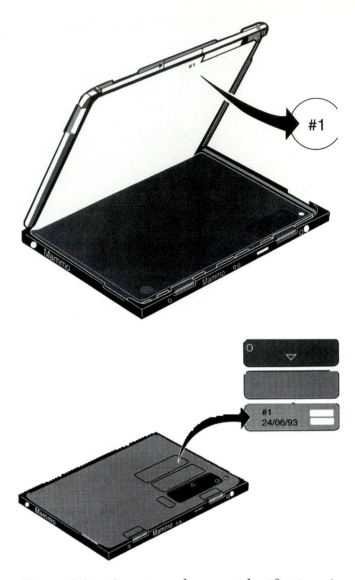

Figure 9.3. Cassette and screen identification. **A.** Inside of screen surface. **B.** Outside of cassette.

Figure 4.11). It is especially important for a facility to *work with the manufacturers* to ensure results comparable to those that the manufacturer(s) says are obtainable.

5.8. Selecting the Appropriate Processor QC Test Tools (Figure 9.4)

A *thermometer* is a device used to measure the temperatures of solutions within the processor. The technologist should not rely on the temperature gauge built into the processor. A mercury thermometer must never be used in a processor, as the mercury is

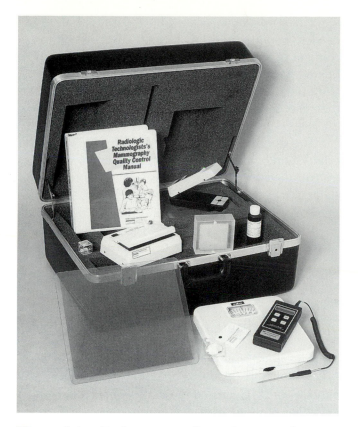

Figure 9.4. Tools necessary for quality-control testing. Courtesy of Nuclear Associates, Carle Place, NY.

a potential contaminant. Glass-type thermometers should be avoided, as they break too easily. A digital thermometer is recommended for mammographic film processors.

The thermometer should have an accuracy of ± 0.3°C or ± 0.5°F. The suggested range is 90 to 100°F.

A *sensitometer* (Figure 9.5A and B) is a device that produces a controlled, repeatable amount of light which is passed through a sensitometric step tablet consisting of 21 graduated steps to produce a series of incremental optical densities on a processed film; this is called a sensitometric control strip. These densities are used to monitor the mid-density or speed index, density difference or contrast index, and the base fog levels.

When using a sensitometer, select the appropriate parameters for the film type that is being used: single versus double and green versus blue.

A *densitometer* (Figure 9.5A and B) consists of a light source and a photo cell for measuring transmitted light. The densities to be read on this unit range from 0.00 to 4.00. This device is used to accurately measure the optical densities used in plotting the

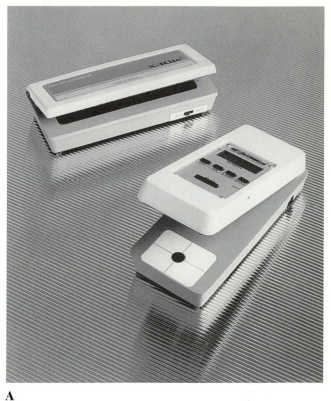

A

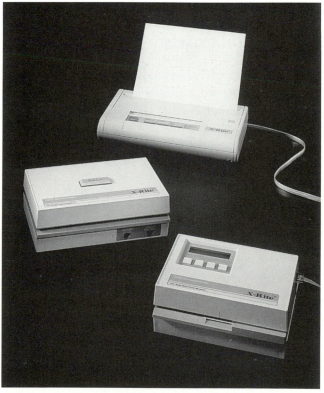

B

Figure 9.5. **A.** Clamshell type of sensitometer and densitometer. **B.** Sensitometer, scanning densitometer, and printer. Courtesy of X-rite Corporation, Grand Rapids, MI.

characteristic curve or the working numerical values such as the mid-density or speed index, the density difference or contrast index, and the base fog levels onto a control chart.

The densitometer will be used for test procedures other than just the PQC; for example, the phantom film.

When beginning a PQC program, select one box of unopened mammography film to be used as the *control box or monitor box of film*. This film must be used for the PQC startup procedure and the daily PQC. One box of the control film will last approximately 3 months when evaluating one processor. Before beginning to use a new control box of film, a crossover procedure must be performed (see Section 9.5).

Upon beginning a QC program, select a *QC cassette*. The cassette can be a one that is used for patient imaging, labeled "QC Cassette" on the back. Or, some facilities may choose to have one cassette designated strictly for QC. Delegating one cassette for QC helps to eliminate additional variables in the QC test results. Use this cassette only for all QC test procedures.

5.9. Control Charts

Each regulatory body normally has its version of control charts designed and available for documenting the data assimilated during the QC testing. The QC control charts usually provide a graphic description of the QC test results. This helps one to quickly visualize trends that may be occurring and thus corrective actions to be taken.

> **Suggestion:** File the QC charts in the QC manual in a calendar format: daily, monthly, semiannually, annually, etc.

5.10. Establishing Operating Levels, Control Limits, and Performance Requirements

Operating levels are those values that one expects when performing the routine QC testing. For example, if, after performing PQC during the 5-day setup period, the average mid-density or speed index is 1.30 for a given film, this is the value that is recorded in the appropriate section of the PQC chart.

The *control limits* are those values that, if exceeded, require additional follow-up tests, either to confirm operator error or if a real problem needs to be investigated immediately. For example, if the control limits for a speed index of 1.30 is ± 0.10 OD, then the highest level accepted is 1.40 and the lowest level is 1.20 OD.

The *performance requirements* are those criteria established by the regulatory body for their expected test result performance. For example, if a regulation states "To determine the mid-density or speed index, select the step on the sensitometric step tablet closest to 1.00 plus base fog," read the various steps until you find the step closest to the prescribed value.

5.11. Viewing Conditions

Viewing conditions in mammography are crucial. Many feel that the term *viewing conditions* refers only the view box, when in fact it refers to the entire area/environment in which the mammogram is reviewed.

All *view boxes* used for viewing mammograms must have identical conditions. It does not help the reader or the technologists to try to obtain satisfactory results when the radiologists are viewing their images on a high-intensity view box but the technologists(s) are using a view box of low intensity. This is discussed in more detail in Section 10.

The *viewing area* implies the environment for reviewing the mammograms: this includes the lighting in the room from overhead lights or from extraneous light and whether masking is used or not.

5.12. Exposure Charts

For every mammography room and for every film-screen combination utilized, a technique chart must be developed and provided.

Exposure charts should include the following:

1. AEC compensation
2. kVp compensation
3. Target and/or filter compensation
4. The implant patient
5. Biopsy tissue samples
6. Unusual position or pathology

5.13. QC Tests for Test Tools (Figure 9.4)

Test tools used for quality control have maintenance of their own to ensure reproducible and consistent results. Consult the manufacturers or their literature for what maintenance is required.

6. Quality Control of Mammography Equipment

The dedicated equipment should be evaluated, at least once a year or as required by government legislation, by a certified physicist or other qualified personnel. Routine preventive maintenance should be performed at least two times a year. Equipment must be evaluated after servicing to ensure that standards are met. Each manufacturer will supply recommendations to meet compliance with major regulatory organizations. Any drift in technique may mean a change in image quality and could mean increased dose to the patient.

6.1. Mammography Unit Evaluation

Screen-film mammography must be performed with a dedicated mammography unit (Chapter 4, Section 1). The target material and filtration of the mammography machine must be appropriate for soft-tissue imaging.

On a routine basis (monthly or as needed) the radiologic technologist should review the mammography equipment. This should include making sure that the locks and lock detentes, the indicator light(s), the compression devices, etc., are all working as designated by the manufacturer.

> Suggestion: Keep a clipboard in the mammography room so that the technologist(s) operating the equipment can make notations if they find something faulty.

On the routine preventive maintenance inspections, the equipment manufacturer should evaluate the mechanical operation of the unit thoroughly. Also, on the annual inspection, the medical physicist should make note of the integrity of the unit.

> Suggestion: Before the HVL is tested, the kVp must be measured for accuracy.

6.2. Half-Value Layer

The half-value layer (HVL) must be evaluated to comply with federal equipment performance standards.

The objective of measuring the HVL is to obtain a mammogram with high contrast and still maintain an acceptable dose to the patient.

At any given kVp setting in the kilovoltage range employed for mammography (below 50), the measured HVL inclusive of the compression device in place must be equal to or greater than the following value (3):

$$HVL \geq kVp/100 + 0.03 \text{ (in mm of aluminum)}$$

Thus, if calculating the HVL at 28 kVp, the HVL must be 0.31 mm of aluminum or greater. If the HVL is greater than 0.39 mm of aluminum at 28 kVp for a Mo/Mo target, the equipment should be serviced. *Note:* This does not exceed federal standards; however, it will affect image quality.

It should be noted that when calculating units with multiple targets and filtration, those evaluating the HVL should consult with the equipment manufacture and/or the regulatory body. In the 1994 ACR manual, it is noted that for these types of units the following is the recommended method of calculation:

$$HVL < kVp/100 + C^* \text{ (mm of aluminum)}$$

*C = constant value of the minimum acceptable HVL

C = 0.12 mm Al for Mo/Mo

C = 0.19 mm Al for Mo/Rh

C = 0.22 mm Al for Rh/Rh

Note: The above is based on an Mo filter thickness of 30 μm or less and Rh filter thickness of 25μm or less.

As units with other target and filtration materials come on the market, consult with the appropriate equipment manufacturer for the above values.

6.3. kVp, mAs, and Timer

To verify that the equipment meets all the standards set, tests should be performed every 6 months. Although not mandatory, repeat tests should be performed upon servicing of the mammography equipment. Standards will be met by testing the following:

1. *kVp accuracy and reproducibility.* Guidelines for recommended tolerances should be checked. As a rule, tolerances are ± 5% from nominal kVp. As seen in Figure 9.6, kVp meters are available to help facilities monitor the kVp of their mammography equipment.
2. *Timer and reproducibility and accuracy.* Guidelines for recommended tolerances should be checked. As a rule, acceptance requires ± 10%.
3. *mAs Linearity and reproducibility.* As a rule, acceptance testing requires ± 10%.
4. *X-ray output reproducibility (R output).* Facilities should know the accepted tolerances. Measurements must be within acceptable limits.

Some QA programs recommend that the above four parameters be evaluated every month. Although this is optimal, some facilities may not have the resources to perform such tests on this schedule. Performing monthly evaluation will pay off in less down time and in maintenance of optimum image quality.

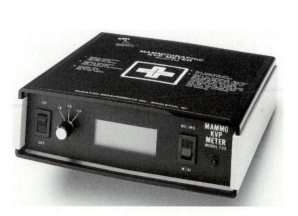

Figure 9.6. Mammographic kVp meter. Courtesy of RMI, Middleton, WI.

6.4. Collimation

Every 6 months or upon servicing the equipment, the collimation must be evaluated. Along the chest wall, the x-ray field extending beyond the image receptor must be no greater than 2% of the SID. The radiation field must not extend beyond any other edge of the image receptor. For equipment that has a dual focal spot, the field size should be checked with both the small and large focal spots. If the equipment provides a visible light field, this should be evaluated to ensure that the light field coincides with the actual x-ray field.

Note: Evaluate the proper alignment of the compression device while evaluating the radiation field alignment. If the compression device does not extend to the end of the image receptor/grid holder, the vertical edge may be visualized. Simultaneously, the compression device should not extend over the edge too far: the suggested tolerance is 1% of the SID (3).

6.5. Focal Spot Size

The size of the focal spot(s) must be evaluated annually with a 0.50 star pattern, a slit camera, a high-contrast resolution pattern, and/or as recommended by the government regulations. Although it is not mandatory, mammography sites that have a large patient volume should have the focal spot checked twice yearly.

Facilities with a dual-focal-spot tube or tubes must have both the large and small focal spots evaluated.

6.6 Automatic Exposure Control

The AEC of the mammography unit must be evaluated for system performance and reproducibility. The newer AEC units have been improved for tracking. *Tracking* refers to the AEC's ability to adjust exposures according to breast thickness and breast tissue composition.

The AEC must be evaluated upon installation of new equipment, upon starting a QC program, upon servicing of the equipment, and at least annually. Adjustments of the AEC may be required if it becomes evident that there has been a "change" on the phantom images. A change on the phantom image may appear as a variation of the image density, thus requiring an increase or decrease in the amount of exposure to obtain the original image density. Tests should also determine the proper response to kVp, mA (when applicable), density, and breast thickness. The QC test on the AEC must demonstrate that the range of the breast sizes and densities encountered in clinical practice are properly imaged (*Note:* Normally reproducibility between 2, 4, and 6 cm is evaluated).

With older equipment, whose AEC has more difficulty tracking, it is strongly advised that an exposure technique chart be developed so that the technologist will know how to alter exposure factors.

Every mammographic unit must have a means of terminating the exposure at the maximum predetermined product of tube current (mA) and exposure time(s). This is referred to as the *backup time.* Tests must be conducted routinely to ensure that the backup timer and the indicator warn the operator that backup has been reached and that these devices are functioning. *Note:* The units that terminate exposure at the beginning of the exposure rather than going to the backup timer also have an audible warning. This warning will notify the technologist to adjust exposure factors.

6.7. Compression

The technologist should routinely check the compression devices to ensure taut, even compression during mammography. Cracks in the compression devices, scratches, weak joints, or loose screws result in uneven compression. Loss of compression will compromise image quality, producing, for example, image blur or an increase in exposure to the patient.

The compression should be checked semiannually with a bathroom scales or other calibrated pressure measurement device (Figure 9.7). The pressure for adequate compression is between 25 to 40 lb. Some government regulations specify that compression must be as high as 55 lb. The compression device must not only have the ability to apply the compression but must also sustain the compression until it is released by the technologist.

Note: When mechanical compression is utilized, the technologist should check to ensure that the tension has not loosened.

Note: Compression must be checked with the C arm in multiple positions. For example, the compression may remain taut for the CC but not the MLO or the 90° lateral projections.

As discussed in Section 5.4 ("Collimation"), the compression device must also be evaluated for cor-

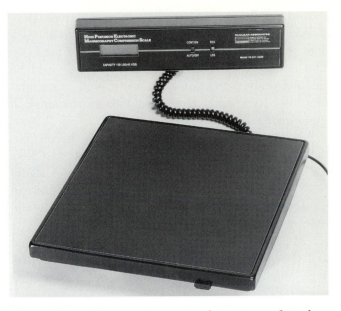

Figure 9.7. Compression test tool. Courtesy of Nuclear Associates, Carle Place, NY.

rect alignment in relation to the image receptor. The compression device, when the appropriate size is selected for the bucky assembly, should exceed the edge of the bucky by 1% of the SID.

The compression device must be cleaned after every patient. Most manufacturers do not recommend the application of alcohol on the compression device. A mild detergent is acceptable for routine cleaning. The infection-control department of the facility should be contacted regarding handling of patients who may have infectious diseases.

7. The Darkroom

The environment in the darkroom must be scrutinized. The darkroom should be used for what it was meant for: loading and unloading of film before and after exposure as well as development. How well the darkroom area is maintained quickly becomes evident on the final mammographic image in terms of dust artifacts on the image or unwanted fog, reducing the overall image quality of the film.

7.1. Darkroom Cleanliness

The darkroom must be kept clean and clear of all debris. All bench tops and feed rays must be kept clear of all foreign material. The mammography darkroom should not be used as a storage area. At no time should anyone smoke or eat in the darkroom. Also note that papers and boxes will cause dust artifacts. The countertops, feed trays, and floor should be cleaned daily. The vents, air ducts, walls, safelight, film bins, pass boxes, etc., should also be cleaned on a routine basis.

At the beginning of each work day, before patients are seen, the darkroom must be cleaned. Clean the countertops and the feed tray with a clean, damp cloth. Then wet mop the floor. This procedure can be done after turning on the processor and while waiting for it to warm up.

Make arrangements with housekeeping to see that the vents (including the door vent) and the top of the safelight are cleaned weekly or on an as-needed basis.

Clean the film bins and pass boxes monthly. When cleaning the film bin, care must be taken to place any unexposed film into a light-tight box. It may be necessary to use a vacuum cleaner to first clean the film bin to remove unwanted paper, etc.

7.2. Checking for Darkroom Fog: Room-Light Leaks or Safelight Problems

Darkroom fog is detrimental to the overall image quality of a mammogram. Fog in the darkroom can be attributed to light leaks or safelight problems.

7.2.1. Checking for Light Leaks

The darkroom should be evaluated for light leaks around the pass boxes, processor, or door. The light, sometimes known as *white light,* may reduce the contrast as well as add to unwanted optical density seen on the mammogram.

1. Go into the darkroom and inspect it. If any obvious cracks or sources of light are seen, correct these immediately.
2. Turn off the lights and close the door. Wait for at least 2 min. Look for leaks around the pass boxes, doors, and any area that may reflect light. Visible light leaks should be eliminated immediately. *Note:* If a phone is installed in the darkroom with a button that lights up when the phone is in operation, cover this light. Also, if a darkroom is

shared with a laser camera, check the lights on the unit.

3. Load a cassette with a sheet of film from an unopened box of film.
4. Take a phantom exposure, exposing the cassette with an exposure factor that results in an optical density between 1.20 and 1.50. (*Note:* Exposed film is more sensitive to light than unexposed film.)
5. Go into the darkroom. Turn out all the lights including the safelight. Close the door.
6. Unload the film, cover one-half of the film. Wait 2 min.
7. Develop the film.
8. If a line is visible on the developed film (see Figure 9.8), the darkroom needs addition lightproofing. Or, an adjacent measurements can be taken with a densitometer of the exposed portion of the image and the covered portion of the image.

The optical density difference should not be greater than 0.05. A darkroom free from light leaks will result in a film with a homogeneous appearance. Evaluate the darkroom semiannually.

7.2.2. Evaluating the Safelight

The safelight must be evaluated upon beginning a QC program and then every 6 months or upon changing either the light bulb or the filter. It is a myth that the filter lasts indefinitely. Several safelight testing

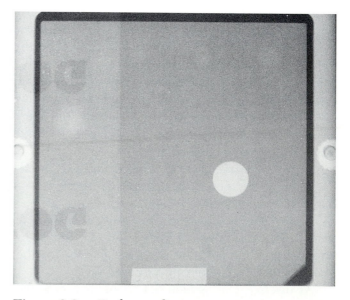

Figure 9.8. Darkroom fog test.

methods and tools are available from most screen or film manufacturers. To evaluate the darkroom safelight, use the procedure above (Section 6.2.1) with one exception. On Step #5, do not turn off the safelight.

As stated in Chapter 4, Section 2, the safelight must be matched to the spectral sensitivity of the film. The most common safelight used is the Kodak GBX filter, with a 7 1/2 to 15-W bulb. The safelight should be placed approximately 4 ft from the work area (confer with the film manufacturer for recommendations).

7.3. Film Storage Bin(s)

The film storage bin, an important component in the darkroom, is taken for granted but can be a source of multiple pitfalls: light leaks, dust, dirt, etc. Often, the film bin is purchased and installed when the darkroom is built. After the initial installation, the film bin is seldom cleaned or checked for light leaks. Here are suggestions for maintaining a film bin properly:

7.3.1. Correct Installation of Film into the Film Bin

Systematically position the film so that it is easy to locate while working in the darkroom. Consider placing the film down into the slots so that the top edge of the film is at an equal height with the dividers or slightly lower.

Care should be taken that the film bin door cannot be "slammed" shut. This has been a cause of pressure artifacts, pinhole-type artifacts, increased static, and an increase in dust and dirt.

Position the film so that the film most commonly used is located closest to the front (nearest the operator) of the bin. Also, position the film so that the film manufacturer's marking notch can be felt for easy identification.

7.3.2. Routine Cleaning

On a regular basis, remove all the film from the film bin. Unexposed film should be placed into an alternative light-tight container/holder. Clean out all the dirt and debris that collects in the bottom of the film bin.

7.3.3 Light Leaks

Fogged edges on unexposed (clear) film may indicate that the film bin is not light-tight. Upon beginning a QC program and when a light leak is suspected, perform the following:

1. In the darkroom, in total darkness, close all open boxes of film in the film bin. Store in a light-tight area.
2. Take a fresh, unexposed piece of film from a newly opened box.
3. Place the film into the film bin. Close the film bin. Make sure that all open film boxes are protected and stored in a light-tight area.
4. Turn on all the white light illumination in the darkroom.
5. Leave the film in the film bin for several hours with the darkroom lights on.
6. Process the film.
7. Inspect the film for fog.

The final image, when inspected, should have no fogging around the edges of the film.

8. The Recording System (Cassette, Screen, and Film)

Poor screen-film contact or a warped cassette will cause image blur. Cassettes and screens should be evaluated at the time of the purchase and every 6 months for optimum screen-film contact. If poor screen-film contact or image blurring is suspected in the interim, a screen-film contact exposure should be taken. The technologist should visually evaluate the screen and cassette for damage when cleaning the screens each day. All cassettes and screens should be labeled with an identification number on both the outside and inside. Then, if a problem occurs, it is easier to isolate the cassette in question.

8.1 Cassette Rotation

To avoid the likelihood of double exposure, a systematic procedure should be established for (a) loading and unloading the cassettes in the darkroom and

(b) separating the exposed and unexposed cassettes. Once the procedure is established, everyone rotating through the mammography section must follow this procedure.

Care must be taken to rotate the cassettes used for patient imaging. In high-volume facilities or a facility utilizing a daylight handling system that is in the mammographic x-ray room, the cassette may not have sufficient time in the "resting" state. In high-volume facilities, it may be more beneficial to have two additional cassettes per size per room to accomplish the rotation. When working with a daylight system, the technologist must take the initiative to rotate the cassettes and not to use the same two cassettes continually simply because it is quicker.

8.2. Cassette-Related Light Leaks

Care must be taken to ensure that the film holder or cassette is correctly closed to avoid light leaks. Before leaving the darkroom, the technologist should feel the edges of the cassette to make sure the cassette is closed. If the hinge or closing mechanism is defective, it must be replaced. Some mammography cassettes have the latch along the chest wall. If the latch is defective, it is not uncommon to find both poor screen-film contact and light leaks.

When light leaks due to the cassette are in question, try the following:

1. Open a new box of film.
2. Load the cassettes in question with the film from the newly opened box.
3. Place the cassette in front of a bank of lighted viewboxes for about 2 to 5 min.
4. Process the film.

If cassette-related light leaks are a problem, there will be black areas on the film.

8.3. Cassette and Screen Cleaning

Cassettes and screens must be cleaned (see Figure 9.9) according to the manufacturer's recommendation. The screen cleaner used must be compatible with the screen in use.

1. It is recommended that screens must be cleaned at least once a week with screen cleaner. This will vary with patient volume, handling, department and darkroom cleanliness, or whenever any arti-

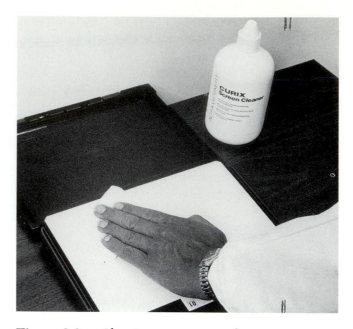

Figure 9.9. Cleaning a mammography cassette.

facts are noticed. The technologist must remember to clean the inside of the cassette cover when cleaning the screen.

> **Suggestion:** Store unused but open packs of cleaning pads in a zip-lock-top type bag to minimize dust accumulation.

2. Many facilities use 4 x 4 in gauze pads. Since mammography cassettes may be cleaned as often as once a day, the gauze may be too rough on the screen surface. A graphic arts product is obtainable from many of the manufacturers that supply your facility with the 4 x 4 inch gauze pads. The graphic arts pad is also 4 x 4 in but is lintless and 100% cotton. Rayon pads are even better if obtainable. Scanner wipes are also excellent, as they contain an antistatic agent. (*Note:* It is essential, whichever product is used for screen cleaning, that "fizzles" or cotton-produced dust artifacts are not created. There are commercial suppliers today who specialize in screen-care products.)
3. Screens must be kept clean of dust. Dust is often attracted by static electricity. The application of an antistatic solution may resolve this problem. In geographic areas of low relative humidity (lower than 40%), a humidifier should be installed. The humidifier must not produce white dust. An air purifier will also help to decrease dust. Both the humidifier and air purifier must have the filters

changed and cleaned monthly or sooner, as required.

Cans of compressed air may also be used to eliminate dust. Care must be taken that the screen does not freeze when the canned air is sprayed onto the screen surface. Follow the directions and do not put the source too close to the screen. Other products available at your local photography shop are:
- Staticmaster brush
- microcleaners
- photowipes
- antistatic cloths

4. The screen surface must be kept dry. After cleaning, cassettes should not be closed until the screens are dry. Closing the cassette before the screen is dry may damage the screen surface, as the film will stick. The cassette should be air-dried upside down with the screen pointed away from the ceiling. Soiling and staining of the screen surface with foreign materials — such as developer, coffee, nail polish, or barium — must be avoided.
5. To prevent dust or dirt from getting in, the cassette must be kept closed. Cassettes must not be left open overnight.
6. Caution should be used in loading and unloading film into a cassette. Care must be taken not to scratch the surface of the screen with jewelry or fingernails.

Points to consider when cleaning screens:

(*Note:* **Do not clean screens and cassettes in the darkroom**).

1. Inspect the area in which you will clean your cassettes. Clean the work area with screen cleaner.
2. Unload the film from the cassettes that you will clean. *Note:* Discard this film. Do not place the film back into the film bin. If the film has attracted any dirt from the cassette, this will be transported into the film bin.
3. Inspect the cassette and screen.
4. Moisten a clean, lint-free cloth with screen-cleaning solution. *Note:* Consider storing the lint-free cloths in a zip-lock-top type bag.
5. Clean the exterior surface of the cassette first.
6. With a new, clean cloth, clean the inside tray of the cassette, paying attention to the corners.
7. With a new, clean cloth, clean the screen.
8. Carefully wipe the screen with the cleaner with even, light strokes from side to side. Overlap the wipes. Clean the entire surface.
9. With a clean, dry, lint-free cloth, dry the screen surface. *Note: The tray as well as the screen must be dry.*
10. Leave the cassette open only long enough to dry. Air-dry upside down.
11. *Do not close the cassette when the screen is damp.*
12. Load the cassette with film and place back into operation.

8.4. Screen Condition and Care

Upon installation, every 6 months, and when image quality is in question, the condition of the screens must be evaluated. An ultraviolet (UV) light (Figure 9.10) can be used to examine the surface of the screen for dirt and pitting. Sometimes screen artifacts are suspected. Determine the source of the artifact and take corrective action. Often artifacts look alike but can be caused by various factors.

Example: The appearance of motion on the image can be caused by:
- uneven compression
- the lack of compression
- patient motion
- poor screen-film contact

Note: Before running out to the local store to buy a UV light, speak with the screen manufacturer. One must purchase a light that produces the same light spectrum as the screen emits. If the two light spectra are not compatible, unnecessary concern may result should something be seen on the screen surface but not visualized on the actual radiograph. The opposite may also occur: something seen on the radiograph may not be seen with the UV light.

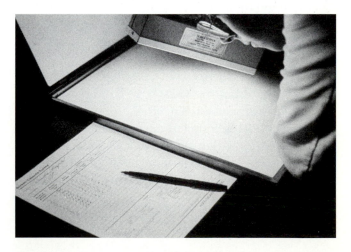

Figure 9.10. Ultraviolet light is used to evaluate a mammography screen.

8.5. Screen-Film Contact

Upon beginning a QC program, every 6 months thereafter or when lack of sharpness is suspected, a screen-film contact image should be taken. To judge screen-film contact, a fine-mesh wire designed for mammography is radiographed (Figure 9.11).

1. The recommended tool for mammography cassettes is a 40-wire-per-inch copper-mesh test tool.
2. Before exposing all the screens and cassettes within a department, unload the film from the cassettes and thoroughly clean the cassettes and screens (see Section 7.3). Inspect all the cassettes to make sure that they are labeled for easy identification, as discussed in Section 5.6.
3. The cassettes should be filled with film at least 15 min before testing to ensure that the trapped air has dissipated.
4. Place the cassette on top of the bucky.
5. The screen-film contact test tool should be placed on top of the cassette (Figure 9.12). (*Note:* Do not put the contact test tool on top of the cassette holder or the bucky. The contact test tool must be placed directly on top of the cassette. Disconnect the bucky when possible, so as to eliminate motion).
6. Move the compression device up as close to the x-ray tube as possible.
7. Select a manual exposure using a kVp between 25 to 28, a mAs value that will give you an exposure time close to 0.5 s. The optical density between the mesh wires along chest wall should be between 0.7 and 0.8. If the film is too dark, it may be necessary to place acrylic sheets on top of the compression device.

Recommendation: Purchase several 1 cm acrylic sheets. During testing use the number of acrylic sheets necessary to meet requirements as stated in point 7.

8. The films are reviewed by standing 3 to 6 ft (1 to 2 m) away from the view box. The areas of poor contact will leave a blurred image and or black spots. Often black spots 1 cm or smaller are caused by dirt. After reviewing the images, if a cassette is in question, repeat the above procedure. If the black spots move, this is caused by dirt or dust.

Common causes for poor screen-film contact are (4):

- dirty or improperly cleaned screens (Figure 9.13)
- warped, damaged, or dented cassettes

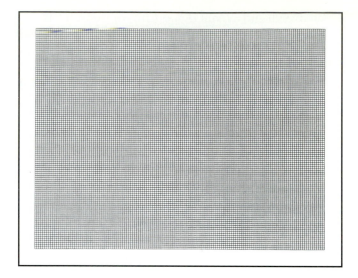

Figure 9.11. Mammography screen-film contact test tool. Courtesy of Nuclear Associates, Carle Place, NY.

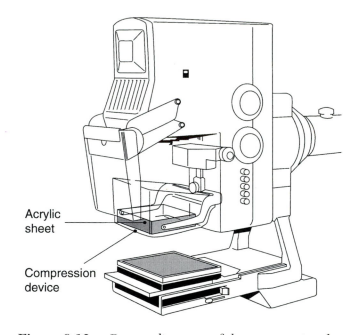

Acrylic sheet

Compression device

Figure 9.12. Proper alignment of the compression device (and acrylic sheet if required), cassette, and screen-film contact test tool.

- warped screens
- trapped air (Figure 9.14)
- improperly mounted screens

8.6. Evaluating Sensitivity of Screens: Screen Speed

Upon beginning a QC program, when replacing a cassette-screen, or annually, all the cassettes and

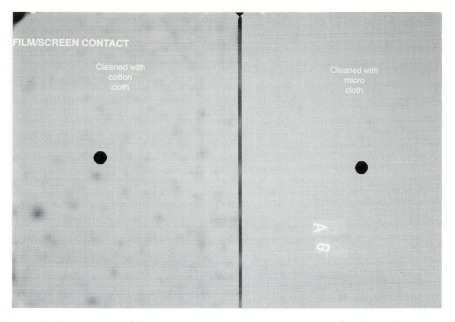

Figure 9.13. Screen-film contact test images. **A.** Improperly cleaned screen. **B.** Properly cleaned screen.

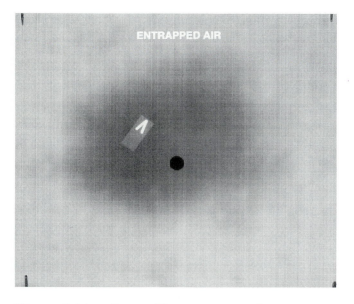

Figure 9.14. Screen-film contact test demonstrating trapped air.

screens must be evaluated for screen speed or sensitivity. In mammography, it is important that all screens produce similar optical densities when exposed. Refer to the regulations for the suggested criteria.

To check the screen speed, examine each cassette by doing the following test procedure (always consult with the regulations to confirm testing methods):

1. Load all the cassette-screens with film taken from an unopened box of film. It is important to use the same emulsion number on all of the exposures to eliminate emulsion variation as a variable. Double check to see that all the cassettes are labeled for easy identification as discussed in Section 5.6.

2. Before exposing the films, the processor and the mammography exposure unit must be operating within limits: the PQC is within limits and the mammography unit is exposing consistently. A good time to schedule this test is after one of the semiannual preventive maintenance (PM) procedures.

3. Place either a phantom, 4.0 cm equivalent cassette size acrylic or BR-12 on top of the bucky-cassette holder. Lower the compression device on top of the phantom selected.

4. Select one of the cassettes, possibly the QC cassette, to be used as the control cassette. *Note:* Check the guidelines being used. Some suggest making three exposures with the control cassette, processing all three films at one time, and then evaluating the optical density. If that density is greater than 0.05, investigate the source of the problem. Others suggest making exposures with the control cassette throughout the test procedure: beginning, midpoint, and end.

5. Select exposure factors that result in an optical density of at least 1.20 or greater.

6. Expose the control cassette. Load all of the cassettes with film from the box of film designated for this test.
7. Expose all the cassettes. Document the mAs per every cassette.
8. Measure the optical density in the center of the phantom.
9. Evaluate the data. The difference between the maximum and minimum of the measured optical densities should match the regulations. For example:

Cassette Number	Optical Density
1 (control cassette)	1.30
2	1.28
3	1.32
4	1.40
5	1.15
6	1.10
7	1.48
8	1.26

If the regulations state that the maximum allowable optical density difference is 0.30 and cassettes #6 and #7 have an optical density difference of 0.38, one can choose to pull cassettes #6 and #7 or cassettes #5 and #6 from operation. Often facilities have more than one mammography room. It is strongly advised that the cassettes in one grouping of values be held in one room, etc. The extreme variations usually occur as a result of replacing a cassette/screen, so the screen number is of a different batch.

One should be aware that it is preferable for mammography cassettes and screens to be replaced more frequently than those in conventional radiography. Some suggest every 2 years. How often the replacement is made generally depends upon the usage; thus, in a low-volume facility, every 2 years may be too often to replace the cassettes and screens. When replacing the cassettes and screens, try to schedule this so that all cassette-screens (or per room) are replaced at one time. This will reduce the chance of extreme variations in speed.

9. Processor Quality Control

Processor QC is the single most important test procedure the technologist can undertake to ensure the most consistent, high-quality mammograms. A film processor can be thought of as the automobile of diagnostic imaging. This "car" is necessary to "drive" the images to their highest quality, but, as with a real automobile, if the least expensive "gasoline" is used and the "oil" or other working parts are never checked, the "car" will finally run so badly that it needs maintenance. To make sure that the film processor always runs well and produces good images, a PQC program must be implemented.

Processor QC is a planned, continuous program of evaluation to ensure that the final images are of consistently high quality. This is accomplished by detecting the photochemical changes in the speed index, contrast index, and fog characteristics of the film before they become visually apparent. A secondary benefit to PQC is the possible detection of potential processing breakdowns before they can result in total loss of operation of the processor.

9.1. Optimizing Processing Conditions

In order to perform PQC properly, the technologist will need some basic equipment: (a) a 21-step sensitometer, (b) a densitometer, and (c) a thermometer (see Section 5.8).

In many facilities, a monthly PM is performed by the local processor service company or by the in-house biomedical staff. Whether a facility has an outside service or in-house service performing the maintenance on the processor, a complete change of chemical solutions and cleaning is mandatory to establish a known optimal level for the processor. Listed in the following sections are the minimum checks that should be performed for a startup PM for PQC.

9.2. Startup Preventive Maintenance

The startup PM procedure should be as follows:

1. Drain and clean developer and fixer tanks and well racks with warm water (no system cleaner).
2. Check developer or fixer crossover rollers for roller wear. Worn or "bumpy" rollers in this area could cause roller artifacts on the film resembling quantum mottle.
3. Fill the fixer tanks with fresh chemical solutions.
4. Fill the developer tank with fresh chemical solutions to ensure that the proper amount of starter solution is added to the tank.
5. Check the recirculation of the developer and fixer

solutions. Poor recirculation of the developer solutions will reduce the developer's ability to fully develop the exposed silver bromide crystals, resulting in loss of density and contrast. Poor recirculation of the fixer solutions will affect the archival quality of the film as well as potentially making the film more sensitive to pinholes in the fixer-to-water crossover racks or in the dryer section.

6. Check and verify the replenishment rates of both the developer and fixer solutions. Inadequate replenishment rates will decrease the solutions' ability to process the film consistently because of slow and gradual exhaustion of the chemicals. The proper replenishment rate for a dedicated mammography processor is usually higher than that of a processor developing conventional film types. Refer to the film manufacturer's recommendations as a guide, based on the chemical brand and overall volume of film per day for the processor.

7. Check and verify the temperature of the developer. Refer to the film manufacturer's recommendation when setting the developer temperature control. After allowing the temperature to stabilize, check the temperature of the developer solutions with a digital thermometer. These types of thermometers can be purchased in most photographic stores. Many processors have temperature gauges built into the units; these may or may not be accurate. Use the hand-held thermometer to check and confirm the processor gauge's accuracy. *Warning:* Do not use a mercury thermometer.

8. Clean the dryer section. Too often the dryer section is ignored. This area can accumulate dust.

A thorough PM is required before staring the PQC program. Preventive maintenance should be done monthly or as required based on the facility's use. Note that monthly PM will reduce processor downtime due to mechanical failure.

9.3. Establishing the Control Limits

In order to properly monitor and evaluate the sensitometric data, it is necessary to establish a baseline standard with upper and lower control limits. These control limits will graphically demonstrate when the processor is out of acceptable range and requires some corrective action. Before beginning the process of establishing the control limits, the facility must refer to the regulatory requirements and procedures.

With a sensitometer, a sensitometric strip should be exposed and processed for 5 consecutive days. Before the strips are processed, the technologist should be sure that these procedures are followed:

1. Warm up the processor for approximately 1 h (consult the processor operator's manual) before running the strip.
2. Run the strip at approximately the same time each day and before radiographing the first patient.
3. Check the developer temperature.
4. Make sure the sensitometer is on (Figure 9.15).
5. Make sure that the sensitometer is matched to the color spectrum of the film being used.
6. Allow a minimum of 10 s between the sensitometer exposures to allow the timer to recycle.
7. Run the sensitometric strip on the same side of the processor to guarantee consistent recirculation agitation on the film.
8. Run the sensitometric strip with the light end leading into the processor to minimize the effects of silver bromide drag on the test strip. Some manufactures may suggest that the step tablet be exposed along the long edge of the film and that side of the film should enter into the processor first. Whichever method is recommended or you choose, continue that method. Varying the method may affect the results.
9. Using the densitometer (calibrate to 0.00 first), read and record the densities of each step on the control strip. At the end of the 5 days, determine the average of the densities for each step.
10. Determine the base plus fog for the 5 days, determine the average, and write this value on the control strip film. (*Note:* Some guidelines sug-

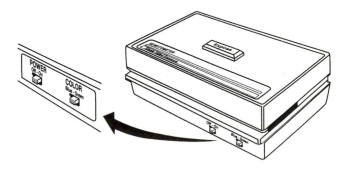

Figure 9.15. To correctly expose film by a sensitometer, turn the sensitometer on and select the appropriate light spectrum.

gest using step 1 of the sensitometric strip to determine the base plus fog. Others suggest measuring base plus fog in an unexposed area of the film.)

11. Based on the 5-day average, determine the mid-density step (often referred to as the speed step, speed index, or speed point). Select the step that has a density closest to 1.20. Identify the step on the sensitometric strip by putting a small mark on it with a felt-tip pen.

12. Based on the 5-day average, determine the density difference (often referred to as the contrast index). To calculate the density difference,
    - Find the step on the sensitometric control strip that measures closes to 2.20. Mark this step on the control strip with a felt-tip pen.
    - Find the step on the control strip that measures closest to but not less than 0.45. Mark this step on the control strip with a felt-tip pen.
    - Subtract the difference between the two steps. Write the difference in the two densities on the control strip.

13. Log the base plus fog, the mid-density (speed index), and the density difference (contrast index) on the appropriate center line on the processor control chart.

14. Identify the upper and lower limits of the base plus fog, the mid-density, and the density difference appropriately on the control chart.

15. The values (numbers) indicated on the control chart will allow for easy plotting and identification of the upper and lower limits on the control chart.

9.4. Daily Processor Quality Control

Each day, before any patients are seen, the PQC must be performed to ensure that the processor is operating within the criteria specified by the QA regulations.

1. Turn on the processor and allow it to warm up.
2. Check the developer temperature.
3. Double check the sensitometer. Select the appropriate color and film settings.
4. With the sensitometer, expose a sheet of film from the control box of film (Figure 9.16).
5. Process the film on the same side of the processor as established.

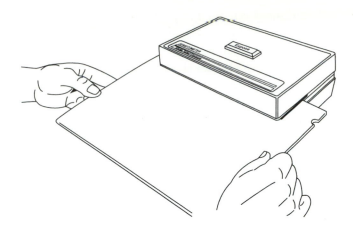

Figure 9.16. Expose a sheet of mammography film with the sensitometer. Remember to place the emulsion side of the film closest to the step tablet (or emulsion side of the film down).

6. Process the film with the light end leading into the processor.
7. Read and record the steps to determine the base plus fog, mid-density, and density difference.
8. Determine whether the density values exceed the control limits. If so, it is important that the test procedure be repeated first to establish that the sensitometric data are accurate and the out-of-limit values are not the cause of the normal variations in the densitometer, sensitometer, and developer temperature fluctuations.
9. Should there still be an out-of-limit reading on the second strip, investigation into its cause will be necessary.

Film manufacturers will provide helpful hints and guides to evaluate the data and possible causes of excessive variations.

Film processor consistency is vital to the production of high-quality mammograms. Without a PQC program performed on a daily basis, variations in image quality can and will occur more frequently, resulting in possible improper diagnosis and unnecessary repeated mammograms. The establishment and maintenance of a PQC program is based on consistency in following the outlined procedures to produce the sensitometric strips. *Variations in procedure can greatly affect the accuracy of the data, resulting in possible unnecessary investigation into false out-of-limit readings.*

9.5. Control-Box Crossover

When a new box of film is opened for PQC, it is important to perform a *crossover* from the old box of film to the new box of film.

Film is produced in batches; thus slight variations in the characteristics in various batches of film will be seen. Also, the storage conditions and the aging characteristics can influence the sensitometric characteristics of film. The purpose of the crossover procedure is to adjust the operating levels on the control chart.

Expose and process five sensitometric strips from each of the old and new boxes of film. Determine the average between each of the three steps as well as the base plus fog from the old and new boxes of film. **The operating levels might have to be adjusted on the control chart for the new levels of the base plus fog, the mid-density (speed index), and the density difference (contrast index).**

The crossover between the old and new boxes should be scheduled to be performed when the chemistry is seasoned. Seasoned chemistry is chemistry that is not fresh or newly mixed but that has had film processed through it.

9.6. Solution Temperatures

Checking the solution temperature is often not included as part of the PQC program. In mammography, depending upon the inherent contrast of the film, temperature variations and shift can become visible. After the temperature has been set for the film type with a given chemistry, processor type, and cycle time, it is wise to occasionally check both the developer and fixer temperatures. *Note:* many QC programs for mammography specify that the developer temperature should be checked daily.

9.7. Replenishment Rates

Replenishment rates are set based upon the type of processor, the chemistry, and the volume of film developed per day as well as the pattern of development. Always consult with the film manufacturer and/or the processor manufacturer as to how to set the correct replenishment rates. *Note:* If there is a change in patient volume or the pattern in which patients are processed, it may be necessary to alter the replenishment rates.

9.8. Analysis of Fixer Retention

In mammography, a woman's examination is her personal "history"; consequently, images are often kept beyond the normal 5 to 7 years for other radiographs. One method to ensure that the films will have acceptable archival quality is to evaluate the fixer retention in the film.

Analysis of the fixer retention in film also permits one to evaluate whether the film is being properly washed in the water tank.

Most film companies recommend that the fixer be analyzed with each new batch of fixer. Some regulations require that this test be done quarterly. The test is quickly done as follows:

1. Develop an unexposed film,
2. Place one drop of the residual hypo test solution on the emulsion side of the film (Figure 9.17).
3. After 2 min, soak up the solution.
4. Then compare the stain on the film to an estimator chart to determine the archival quality of the film, the washing capabilities of the processor, and how much fixer is being retained.

9.9. Processor Maintenance

Establish a routine processor maintenance program for your processor. Most facilities have a program in place for all processors on a monthly basis. For mammography, this should be no different. Much of what

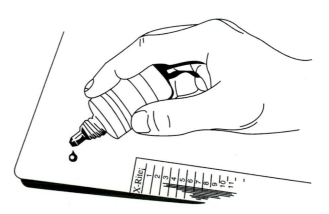

Figure 9.17. Place one drop of hypo test solution onto the emulsion side of the film to determine the archival quality of the film.

was pointed out in Section 7.3 is what is evaluated by the maintenance personnel.

Ask how to keep the processor clean. For example, which rollers should be rinsed every day?

A reminder: Too often the dryer is not cleaned! Dust and dirt that builds up in the dryer may be the cause of pick-off!

In your routine processor maintenance, include a routine program for the chemistry mixer. Too often the mixer is overlooked. Ensure that the float is correctly set to mix the chemistry as desired. Hoses should be checked for kinks that may inhibit replenishment of the chemistry. Does the water enter into the mixer at the right time and the correct dilution? Is the mixer providing accurate mixing of the solution?

If you have a chemistry solutions company bringing in the chemistry premixed, the barrels that hold the solution should be cleaned on a regular basis. The hoses should be checked.

9.9.1. Daylight Systems

The processors will be quality-controlled and maintained in the same fashion as a darkroom processor (unless otherwise indicated by the manufacturer). Speak to the manufacturer about suggestions for maintaining the transport section and the film magazines.

> Suggestions:
> 1. Clean the transport sections quarterly (or as recommended by the manufacturer).
>
> 2. Clean the magazine each time a new box of film is placed into the magazine or film holder. Often chips of film or dust will accumulate in the magazine.

9.10. Batch Processing

Facilities that batch-process their case load—whether mobile or screening facilities—must perform PQC before beginning to develop the exposed stored films.

One concern when batch processing is employed is *latent image fading*. An exposed film in which the processing is postponed for an extended period of time may produce an image with lower optical density as compared with film that is processed immedi-

ately. This effect, latent image fading, is caused by the instability of the latent image.

If batch processing is employed, contact the film manufacturer to obtain the data on the effects of latent image fading on the film. Time delays of film may affect both the speed and the contrast. To minimize the effect of latent image fading, try to arrange the schedule so that the collected films are processed as consistently as possible. When necessary, exposure factors must be adjusted accordingly.

10. The Viewing Conditions

Often overlooked in obtaining optimum image quality in mammography are the viewing conditions. It is not uncommon to find that not only do all the view boxes within a department vary in intensity and color but that the actual viewing environment is vastly different. It is imperative to have uniform viewing conditions for the technologist(s) and the radiologist(s). Quality-control procedures must be an integral part of ensuring that optimal viewing conditions are maintained.

10.1. Cleaning Procedures for the View Boxes

On a routine basis (weekly is suggested), do the following:

1. Inspect the viewboxes.
   - The surface of the view box should provide uniform brightness.
   - The lamps must have the same color as all the view boxes used to read mammograms.
2. Clean the view boxes using a glass cleaner such as Windex and soft paper towels, and remove all marks—for example, wax-pencil marks.
3. Clean the magnification glasses.
4. Make sure the masking material is easily available.

Twice a year, the insides of the view boxes should be cleaned. The power should be disconnected before cleaning.

10.2. Measurement of Luminance, Color, and Illuminance

Annually, unless the need arises sooner, both the luminance and color as well as the illuminance of the viewing area must be evaluated with a photographic exposure meter (Figure 9.18).

10.2.1. Luminance

View-box intensity measurements are made by placing the photographic exposure meter near the surface of the view box. Excluding all extraneous light (turn off all overhead lights, etc.). Measure several points over the surface of the view box except the edge.

The suggested luminance for a mammography viewbox is 3500 nit.

10.2.2. Color or Spectrum of the View Box

The color emitted by the bulbs of the view box influences the look of the mammogram also. The lower or cooler color temperatures give the mammogram a "warmer" appearance; conversely the higher color temperatures result in a "cool" appearance. The cooler appearance is usually preferred in mammography, as it produces an appearance toward the direction of the blue tones.

To date, specifications are not available for the color temperature of the view boxes.

10.2.3. Illuminance

The ambient light can also be measured with a photographic exposure meter. Before making the measurements, adapt the viewing conditions so that they replicate the "normal" working conditions. For example, if there is a window in reading area, is the curtain open or closed? Are the overhead lights on or off? Second, turn on the view boxes. Place the light meter parallel to the view box with the diffuser surface pointed away from the view box.

The suggested room ambient lumination level is < 50 lux (see Section 9.2). (*Note:* Confer with regulator requirements and the exact method how to evaluate the viewing conditions. For example, in the European guidelines the illuminance criterion is < 10 lux; however, the view boxes are turned off when the measurements are taken. In North America, the regulations suggest < 50 lux, and the view boxes are turned on when the measurements are taken.)

10.2.4. Miscellaneous Suggested Performance

At all times unexposed areas of film must be masked to reduce the extraneous light.

The suggested frequency for replacing fluorescent tubes within the view boxes is every 18 to 24 months. It is strongly recommended that all tubes be replaced at one time to avoid uneven brightness.

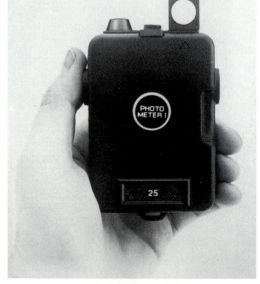

Figure 9.18. EV exposure meter. Courtesy of Nuclear Associates, Carle Place, NY.

11. Evaluating the Entire Imaging Chain

In this section, those QC actions taken to review the entire imaging chain are defined. These include (a) phantom imaging, (b) patient exposure or dose, (c) artifact analysis, and (d) retake analysis.

11.1. Phantom Imaging

There are several commercially available mammography detail phantoms. These phantoms are designed to evaluate the system's ability to image structures similar to those found clinically. Before purchasing a phantom, it is important to establish which phantom has been chosen by the facility's regulatory organization.

Upon beginning a QC program or installing new mammography equipment, a "standard" or reference phantom image must be taken and kept on file. As required by the QA program (weekly or monthly) or on an as-needed basis, a phantom image should be taken to evaluate and record image quality. The reference phantom image permits a quick check to compare the subsequent images, looking for potential changes. Every time the mammographic equipment is recalibrated, a reference phantom must be reestablished.

It is strongly suggested that the reference phantom be taken not only after the mammography equipment has been calibrated but also after preventive maintenance of the processor with fresh chemistry. One may consider exposing future phantom testing in conjunction with the processor PM and chemistry cycle.

Most mammography phantoms have a grading sheet to help the reader score the phantom image. The same individual should always evaluate the phantom image on the same view box each time.

Changes in the phantom image may be perceived as a loss in resolution. For example, on the most recently exposed phantom film, a variation in optical density may be seen. This may be caused by an inconsistent power source, a drop in the mA or kVp, a change of film emulsion number, or a reaction resulting from the activity of the chemistry in the processor. By exposing the phantom daily with an AEC exposure, noting the mAs, and measuring the optical density of the film, the technologist can quickly determine before imaging the first patient how the entire imaging chain is performing and what if any corrections must be made in exposure techniques. It is important always to take the phantom film with the same cassette. This cassette should be marked "QC."

For the purposes of discussion, reference is made to the RMI 156 (Figure 9.19). Most phantoms used in the various QC programs, like the RMI 156 phantom, are made of acrylic blocks and are equal to a compressed breast (4.5 cm) in thickness. The RMI

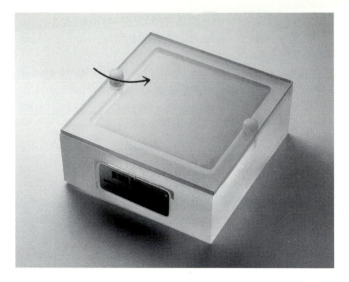

Figure 9.19. RMI Phantom 156. Courtesy of RMI, Middleton, WI.

156 phantom contains a wax insert with five sets of aluminum oxide specs to simulate microcalcifications. There are six different-sized nylon fibers to simulate fibrous structures and five different-sized simulated tumor masses (Figure 9.20). (*Note:* As of June 1990, an identification number has been imbedded into the wax insert.)

The various-sized objects within the RMI 156 phantom are as follows:

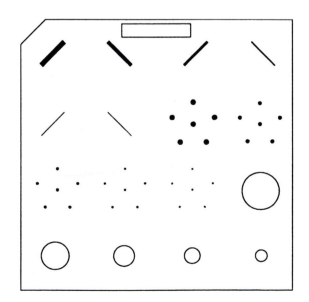

Figure 9.20. Line drawing of the objects imbedded into the pink wax insert in an accreditation phantom. Courtesy of Nuclear Associates, Carle Place, NY.

Fibers (mm)	Masses (mm)	Specks (mm)
1.56	2.00	0.54
1.12	1.00	0.40
0.89	0.75*	0.32*
0.75*	0.50	0.24
0.54	0.25	0.16
0.40		

* To be accepted by the ACR MAP accreditation program, the minimum imaging system must detect a 0.75-mm fiber, 0.32-mm speck, and a 0.75-mm mass (2).

To expose a phantom properly, one should:
1. Place the phantom on top of the image receptor. (*Note:* Most phantoms on the market have a chest-wall side and a nipple side. Position the phantom on the image receptor as instructed by the manufacture and or the regulations.) See Figure 9.21.
   • The pink wax insert must face the x-ray tube, not the cassette holder.
   • The phantom is marked to indicate the nipple side of the phantom.
   • The chest wall edge of the phantom is placed flush with the chest wall edge of the cassette holder.
   • Place the 4-mm disk on top of the phantom and position the disk so that the objects are not obscured. Each time the phantom image is taken,

the disk should be placed in a consistent position.
2. Lightly place the compression device on top of the phantom.
3. Place the film and cassette in the image receptor.
4. Expose the phantom.
   • Select an exposure required to provide a 4.5-cm compressed breast. The regulations will indicate the desired optical density for evaluation.
   • Select the kVp used in clinical applications unless otherwise specified.
   • If the AEC is used, move the photo-cell detector under the pink wax insert.
   • Document the recorded mAs.
5. Evaluate the phantom image. Refer to the regulations for performance criteria. Take appropriate corrective action as needed.

Note: Once the correct method for exposing the phantom has been established, it is important to repeat all phantom films in the same manner. Consistency is the key to success.

> **Suggestion:** After loading the film into the QC cassette, wait 15 min before taking the exposure. If there is any entrapped air in the cassette, it may minimize the number of objects that can be visualized.

11.2. Patient Exposure, Dose

Annually or upon adjusting or servicing of x-ray equipment, patient entrance exposure measurements must be taken. The dose delivered during a mammogram should not exceed government standards or regulations for the average 4.5-cm compressed breast. The ACR recommends that the average glandular dose be no greater than 0.3 rads per view.

The procedure for measuring radiation dose acts as a "checks and balances" on the quality of the entire imaging chain. A well-established quality assurance program will assist in maintaining the lowest exposure for the patient. The major factors that affect the dose are:

• imaging chain
• x-ray beam energy
• compression
• patient's breast tissue type (composition) and thickness

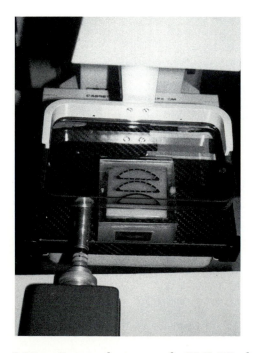

Figure 9.21. Proper placement of a RMI 156 phantom on the image receptor. Note the dosimeter adjacent to the phantom.

1. *Imaging chain:* The imaging chain refers to the equipment, the screen-film combination, and the processing environment. The optimized imaging system will result in lower exposures, thus resulting in a lower dose to the patient.

2. *X-ray beam energy:* The higher the kVp and the half-value layer (HVL), the lower the patient dose. It is important, however, to remember not to increase kVp or HVL just to decrease exposure to a point where the diagnostic quality is lost.

3. *Compression:* At all times compression of the breast tissue should be taut unless the patient's condition warrants otherwise. In such a situation, the inability to compress the breast should be documented on the history form. Greater compression will result in a decrease in exposure, which will result in decreased dose to the patient (see Chapter 6, Section 1).

4. *Patient's breast tissue type and thickness:* The patient's breast tissue type and the thickness of the breast will also affect the amount of exposure necessary to produce a predetermined image density (see Chapter 6).

Several terms (5) often used in discussing dose must be defined.

1. The *skin dose* is the actual x-ray exposure to the skin. The skin dose is the most often quoted as it is the easiest to calculate.

2. The *entrance dose* is the dose delivered in air. It is measured at the bottom of the compression device.

3. The *absorbed dose* is the average dose to the entire breast. One cannot measure the dose inside the breast. The absorbed dose is calculated and estimated by measuring the x-ray exposure with a given phantom and knowing the HVL, the breast tissue type, and the thickness of the breast.

4. The *average glandular dose,* the most important in mammography, is the average dose to the entire breast.

5. *Dosimetry* is the science of measurement of the intensity of the radiation.

6. *Dosimeters* are the devices used to measure radiation.

The dose is usually measured in one of two ways:

1. Thermoluminescent dosimeters (TLD)
2. Ionization chamber

A TLD is a convenient type of dosimeter that absorbs radiation energy, allowing later measurements with laboratory instruments. A small strip is applied to the patient or phantom during exposure. The exposed strip is then returned to the supplier for processing and evaluation.

The ionization chamber is a device for measuring exposure by recording the radiation produced in air for a given exposure factor. The ionization chamber is placed next to the phantom or the patient during exposure or on top of the image receptor. Most mammography facilities do not have an ionization chamber unless they have an in-house physicist or a biomedical department.

Dose evaluations should be executed the same way as the routine imaging of a patient. If the AEC is used, a patient entrance exposure measurement can be made by placing a 4.5-cm acrylic breast phantom over the photo cell. The probe of a dosimeter is positioned adjacent to the phantom at the skin entrance level (Figure 9.21). The exposure factors should be set for the average 4.5-cm compressed breast.

When necessary, the mammography equipment service can place a mAs meter or elapsed exposure time indicator (Figure 9.22) on the unit. Newer mammography units have mAs readout meters that will record exposure factors. A manual setting versus an AEC setting should be selected for measuring the

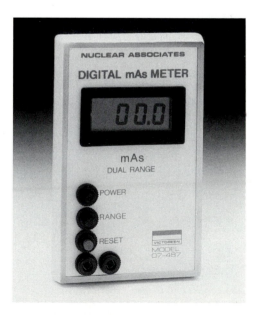

Figure 9.22. Digital mAs meter that can be attached to any mammography machine.

10

Troubleshooting Guide

This chapter discusses problems you may encounter while performing a mammogram and their likely solutions. If you are having difficulty achieving the desired results, for example, in positioning, refer to the appropriate troubleshooting guide. Several of the troubleshooting guides are excerpts from booklets manufacturers have supplied.

1. Troubleshooting the Radiographic System: Symptoms and Possible Causes (Reprinted courtesy of Agfa Corporation, Ridgefield Park, NJ)
2. Diagnosing and Resolving Processor-Related Artifacts (Reprinted courtesy of Du Pont Medical Products, Wilmington, Del.)
3. Guide to Common Processing Problems—Non–Du Pont Chemistries (Reprinted courtesy of Du Pont Medical Products, Wilmington, Del.)
4. How to Alter Exposure Factors
5. Positioning Problems
6. Parameters to Be Tested for Good Mammography Quality Assurance

1. Troubleshooting the Radiographic System: Symptoms and Possible Causes

Low Density

A. Underexposure

1. Wrong Exposure factors
   a. Too low kilovoltage
   b. Too low milliamperage
   c. Too short exposure
   d. Too great focal-film distance
2. Meters out of calibration
3. Timer out of calibration
4. Inaccurate setting of meters or timer
5. Drop in incoming line voltage
   a. Elevators, welders, furnaces, blowers, etc., on same circuit
   b. Insufficient size of power line or transformers
6. Photocell timer out of adjustment
7. Incorrect centering of patient to photocell
8. Central ray of X-ray tube not directed on film
   a. X-ray tube rotated in casing
9. Distance out of grid radius
10. Bucky timer inaccurate
11. One or more valve tubes burned out. (Full wave rectifying machines)

B. Underdevelopment

1. Improper development
   a. Time too short
   b. Temperature too low (hydroquinone inactive below 55°F, 13°C)
   c. Combination of both
   d. Inaccurate thermometer
2. Exhausted developer
   a. Chemical activity used up
   b. Activity destroyed by contamination
3. Diluted developer
   a. Water overflowed from wash tank
   b. Insufficient chemical mixed originally due to tank being larger than rating
   c. Improper additions
4. Incorrectly mixed developer
   a. Exact capacity of tank
   b. Mixing ingredients in wrong sequence
   c. Omission of ingredient
   d. Unbalanced formula composition

High Density

A. Overexposure

1. Wrong exposure factors
   a. Too high kilovoltage
   b. Too high milliamperage
   c. Too long exposure
   d. Too short focal-film distance
2. Meters out of calibration
3. Timer out of calibration
4. Inaccurate setting of meters or time
5. Surge in incoming line voltage
6. Photocell timer out of adjustment
7. Incorrect centering of patient to photocell

B. Improper development

1. Time too long
2. Temperature too high
3. Combination of both
4. Inaccurate thermometer
5. Insufficient dilution of concentrated developer
6. Omission of bromide when mixing

C. Fog—see section on fog

1. Light-struck
2. Radiation

3. Chemical
4. Film deterioration

Low Contrast

A. Overpenetration from too high kilovoltage

1. Overmeasurement of part to be examined
2. Incorrect estimate of material or tissue density
3. Meters out of calibration
4. Meters inaccurately set
5. Surge in incoming line voltage
6. Undermeasurement of focal-film distance

B. Scattered radiation

1. Failure to use Bucky diaphragm
2. Failure to use stationary grid
3. Failure to use cutout diaphragm
4. Failure to use suitable cones
5. Failure to use lead backing cassette

C. Too short exposure

1. Timer out of calibration
2. Timer inaccurately set
3. Overload relay kicked out

High Contrast

A. Underpenetration from too low kilovoltage

1. Undermeasurement of part to be examined
2. In parts of varying thicknesses, setting of kilovoltage for thinner sections
3. Meters out of calibration
4. Meters inaccurately set
5. Drop in incoming line voltage
   a. Elevators, welders, furnaces, etc., on same line
   b. Insufficient size of power line or transformer
6. Overmeasurement of focal-film distance

B. Too long exposure

1. Timer out of calibration
2. Timer inaccurately set

C. Improper development

Fog

A. Unsafe light

1. Light leaks into processing room
   a. Leaks through doors, windows, etc.
   b. Poorly designed labyrinth entrance
      (1) Bright light at outer entrance
      (2) Reflection from white uniforms of persons passing through
   c. Sparking of motors
      (1) Ventilating fans
      (2) Drier fans
      (3) Mixer-barium
      (4) Light leaks in film-carrying box
2. Safelights
   a. Bulb too bright
   b. Improper filter
      (1) Not dense enough
      (2) Cracked
      (3) Bleached
      (4) Shrunken
3. Luminous clock and watch faces
4. Lighting matches in darkroom
5. Where film is carried from machine to darkroom in containers, container may leak light

B. Radiation

1. Insufficient protection
   a. During delivery or transportation in laboratory or shop
   b. Film storage bin
   c. Loaded cassette racks—steel back should face toward source or radiation
   d. For loading darkroom
2. Improper storage
   a. Radium
   b. Isotopes
   c. X-ray machines

C. Chemical

1. Prolonged development (see B, 1., 2., 3. under "High density")
2. Developer contaminated
   a. Foreign matter of any kind (metals, etc.)
3. Contaminated solutions

D. Deterioration of film

1. Age (use oldest film first)

2. Storage conditions
   a. Too high temperatures
      (1) Hot room
      (2) Cool room, but near radiator or hot pipe
   b. Too high humidity
      (1) Damp room
      (2) Moist air
      (3) Ammonia or other fumes present in darkroom or other work area
3. Delivery conditions
   a. Moisture precipitation when cold box of film is opened in hot, humid room (fresh boxes should be stored overnight at room temperature before opening)

E. Excessive pressure on emulsions of unprocessed film

1. During storage
2. During manipulation in darkroom

F. Loaded cassettes stored near heat, sunlight, or radiation

Stains on Radiographs

A. Yellow

1. Exhausted, oxidized developer
   a. Old
   b. Covers left off
   c. Scum on developer surface
      (1) Oil from pipelines
      (2) Impure water used when mixing
      (3) Dust
2. Prolonged development
3. Insufficient rinsing
4. Exhausted fixing bath

B. Dichroic

1. Old, exhausted developer
   a. Colloidal metallic silver
2. Nearly exhausted fixer
3. Developer containing small amounts of fixer or scum
4. Films partially fixed in weak fixer, exposed to light and refixed
5. Prolonged intermediate rinse in contaminated water

C. Green-tinted

1. Insufficient fixing or washing

Deposits on Radiographs

A. Metallic

1. Oxidized products from developer
2. Silver salts reacting with hydrogen sulfide in air to form silver sulfide
3. Silver-loaded fixer

B. White or crystalline

1. Milky fixer
   a. Hardener portion added too fast while mixing
   b. Hardener portion added when too hot
   c. Excessive acidity
   d. Developer splashed into fixer
   e. Insufficient rinsing
2. Prolonged washing

C. Grit

1. Dirty water
2. Dirt in dryer

Marks on Emulsion Surfaces

A. Runs

1. Insufficient fixing
   a. Weakened fixer
   b. Unbalanced formula
   c. Exhausted ingredients
   d. Low acid content
      (1) Deficient when fresh
      (2) Diluted from rinse water
      (3) Neutralized by developer because of insufficient or no rinsing
2. Drying temperature too high
3. Contact with hot viewing box

B. Blisters

1. Formation of gas bubbles in gelatin
   a. Carbonate of developer reacting with acid of fixer

   b. Unbalanced processing temperatures
      (1) Combination of hot fixer and cool developer
      (2) Combination of cool fixer and hot developer
   c. Excessive acidity of fixer
   d. No agitation of film when first placed in fixer

C. Reticulation

1. Nonuniform processing temperatures
   a. Developer (hot)
   b. Fixer (cool)
   c. Wash
2. Weakened fixer with little hardening action

D. Frilling

1. Weakened fixer with little hardening action
2. Hot processing solutions
   a. Developer
   b. Fixer
   c. Wash

E. Drying marks from uneven drying of gelatin

1. Excessive drying temperatures
2. Extremely low humidity
3. Puddies (buckshot marks)
   a. Drops of water striking semidried emulsion surface
4. Streaks
   a. Drops of water running down semidried emulsion surface
      (1) Water splashes
      (2) Drying air flow too rapid
      (3) Insufficient or uneven squeeze from last roller pair in water rack

F. White spots

1. Screens pitted
2. Grit or dust present on film or screens
3. Chemical dust settling on films or screens (particles of certain chemical dusts will also cause black spots)

G. Artifacts

1. Crescents—-rough handling
2. Smudgemarks—-fingerprints or finger abrasions
3. Bands in marginal area usually due to screen mounting medium.

Slow Drying

A. Waterlogged films

1. Insufficient *hardening* in fixer
   a. Too short fixing period
   b. Weakened fixer from splashing
   c. Exhausted fixer
   d. Insufficient acidity (carryover developer, fixer)
   e. Wash water too warm

B. Incoming air too humid

C. Incoming air too cold

D. Air velocity too low

Streaks on Radiographs

A. Insufficient agitation while processing

B. Fog

C. Chemically active deposits (dried chemicals)

D. Pressure fog

E. Scratches

1. Careless handling
2. Grit present in air, in cassettes, or on illuminator

F. Exposure to white light before complete fixing

G. Uneven drying due to high temperature and low humidity

Lack of Detail or Fuzziness

A. Motion (tube, film, subject)

1. Inadequate immobilization
2. Too long exposure
3. Vibration of floor
4. Slipping of subject on mount
5. Stepping on and off operator's platform during exposure where control and tube are mounted on common mobile base
6. Failure to arrest tube vibration after positioning before making exposure

B. Poor contact of intensifying screens

C. Improper distance relationship

1. Object film distance too great
2. Target film distance too short

D. Improper focal spot

1. Too large
2. Damaged (cracked or pitted)

Static

A. Low humidity

B. Insulation

1. Use of rubber gloves, shoes, finger cots, etc.
2. Insulated flooring

C. Improper handling in

1. Removal from box
2. Removal from interleaving paper
3. Loading cassette
4. Unloading cassette
5. Loading hanger
6. Films stacked before processing

2. Diagnosing and Resolving Processor-Related Artifacts

tinues to improve and makes further demands for optimum processing conditions.

William R. Mannia
Jean E. Bartlett

Introduction

The attached information was tabulated for use by sales and service personnel to resolve processor-related problems associated with new film technology.

Many processors found in the marketplace today are not designed to handle the higher-resolution, single-emulsion films used more and more frequently. But with minor modifications, most processors, when properly maintained, can be adjusted to produce high-quality, artifact-free radiographs.

The artifacts listed in this booklet are limited to those caused by design deficiencies or improper maintenance; the processors are those that were actually worked on to resolve a film concern. This booklet will be updated and expanded as the number of competitive processors increases and as film technology con-

Important

Verify that the problem is with all emulsions and not caused by a defect associated with one emulsion number. To do this, process films of more than one emulsion number; a density of 0.8 to 1.8 will normally show the artifacts. Process single-emulsion films both emulsion up and emulsion down. Most plus-density artifacts are caused by the developer rack.

Note:

Plus Density Mottle/Lines—When developer racks cannot be totally submerged in cleaning solution, they will require a thorough cleaning with a nonabrasive pad, such as a 3M Scotch-Brite® pad. If the racks are only flushed with a systems cleaner and rinsed, emulsion will build up on the hard plastic rollers within two weeks.

COMMON PROCESSING-RELATED ARTIFACTS

Processors with Problems: Film Types Affected

Artifact	M6B	M6AN M6AW	M8	M7	M35	DDP	QC1 R/T	QC1	PAKO 14X	KONICA QX400
A — Buff Mark (°)	All	#All	#All	#All	All	All	—	—	—	—
B — Pi Line (°)	All	#All	#All	#All	All	All	—	—	—	—
C — Multiple Bands (°)	All	#All	#All	#All	All	—	(1)	—	—	—
D — Black Spots (°)	—	—	All	—	—	—	—	All	—	—
E — Mottle/Lines (°)										
— Random	(1)	(1)	(1)	(1)	(1)	—	—	—	—	—
— Repetitive	(1)	(1)	(1)	(1)	(1)	—	—	—	—	(1)
F — Curtain Runback	(2)	(2)	(2)	(2)	(2)	—	—	—	—	—
G — Water Spots	—	—	—	—	—	All	—	—	All	—
H — White Blotches/ Black Rings	(3)	(3)	(3)	(3)	(3)	(3)	(3)	(3)	(3)	(3)
I — Pickoff	(1)	(1)	(1)	(1)	(1)	(1)	(1)	(1)	(1)	—

Key: All = Any single- or double-emulsion x-ray film.
    (1) = Mammography and video films.
    (2) = Some tabular grain films, mammography and video films.
    (3) = Mammography films (artifacts seen on Kodak and Du Pont processors).
    (°) = Some tabular grain films will not normally have this problem.
  #All = The processors usually will not show the problem unless the developer rack was rebuilt during or after 1988.

Recommended Solutions

Artifact Definitions
A. *Buff Mark:* A definite line positioned 1 5/8 in from the leading edge of the film. Noticeable on exposed or unexposed films, it shows only on single-emulsion films that are fed into the processor emulsion down. The mark does not appear on many of the tabular grain products.

B. *Pi Line:* One or more lines on the film at 3 1/8 in intervals. The first line will be 3 1/8 in from the leading edge of the film. If there is more than one line

Processor Modifications to Reduce or Eliminate Problems

	Recommended Solutions									
Artifact	M6B	M6AN M6AW	M8	M7	M35	DDP	QC1 R/T	QC1	PAKO 14X	KONICA QX400
A — Buff Mark	A1	A1	A1	A1	A1	A2	—	—	—	—
B — Pi Line	A1	A1	A1	A1	A1	B1	—	—	—	—
C — Multiple Bands	C1	C1	C1	C1	C1	C1	C1B	—	—	—
D — Black Spots	—	—	D1	—	—	—	—	D1	—	—
E — Mottle Lines										
— Random	E1	E2	E2	E2	E1	—	—	—	—	—
— Repetitive	E3	E3	E3	E3	E3	—	—	—	—	E4
F — Curtain Runback	F2	F1	F1	F1	F2	—	—	—	—	—
G — Water Spots	—	—	—	—	—	G2	—	—	G1	—
H — White Blotches/ Black Rings	H1	H1	H1	H1	H1	H1	H1	H1	H1	—
I — Pickoff	I1	I1	I1	I1	I1	I1	I2	I2	I1	—

Success Rate

A — Buff Mark
- A1: Should totally eliminate the problem.
- A2: Should reduce the artifact to an acceptable level; however, it may reappear after the next cleaning. Often, the guides are moved during cleaning and will need adjustment.

B — Pi Line
- A1: May reduce the artifact.
- B1: Will reduce the artifact.

C — Multiple Bands
- C1: Should eliminate the problem with double-emulsion films and reduce the artifacts on single-emulsion film to an acceptable level.
- C1B: Will eliminate the problem.

D — Black Spots
- D1: Will eliminate the problem.

E — Mottle/Lines
- E1: Will eliminate the problem.
- E2: Will reduce the problem to an acceptable level.
- E3: Will reduce the problem to an acceptable level.
- E4: Will eliminate the problem.

F — Curtain Runback
- F1: Will reduce the problem.
- F2: Will reduce the problem.

G — Water Spots
- G1: Will eliminate the problem.
- G2: Will eliminate the problem.

H — White Blotches
- H1: Will eliminate the problem.

I — Pickoff
- I1: Will eliminate the problem.
- I2: Will eliminate the problem.

on the film, the density should be less with each line. The line will not extend to the edge of the film.

C. Multiple Bands: Plus-density lines that are parallel to the leading edge of the film and are seen only on exposed films. The lines, which can vary in width and distance, appear on both sides of the film. Sometimes, they are worse on one side. They are easily seen with image densities between 0.8 and 2.0. This is a processor problem caused by swollen shafts and bearings in the "D" roller Kodak processors.

D. Black Spots: Plus-density spots found throughout exposed and unexposed films. They appear as crescents when viewed with a 10X magnifier. In most cases, these spots are caused by excessive pressure form processor parts, such as worn bearings, gears, and shafts.

E. Mottle/Lines: Plus-density patterns, appearing as background noise, that are only found on exposed films. The patterns are easily seen between densities of 0.8 and 2.0. In some cases, the pattern can appear as coarse lines diagonal to the film edges. In other cases, the lines are very fine and run parallel to the leading edge of the film. These lines can be caused by worn, damaged, or defective rollers. Often, the developer rollers are covered with emulsion because they were just rinsed off rather than being thoroughly cleaned.

F. Curtain Runback: Plus-density, nonuniform pattern on the trailing edge of the film. In extreme cases, the pattern looks like liquid flowing over the film. However, it usually appears as a plus-density blob along the trailing edge. The pattern can extend between 1 in and 2 in from the film edge and may repeat anywhere on the film in extreme cases.

G. Water Spots: Plus- and minus-density blotches spread throughout the image area and found only on exposed films. The blotches may change from plus-density to minus-density across the same film. To date, this problem has been seen only with Pako (AFP) 14XL or 14X processors.

H. White Blotches: Minus-density areas that are found anywhere across the film. They do not appear in any pattern and are related to the film. They can be very large and nonuniform in size. They are visible at any density but only on exposed films. Sometimes, black rings appear in the lower-density areas of the film. To date, these blotches have only been found on mammography films.

I. Pick-off: The removal of emulsion from the film base during processing. The area where the emulsion is removed appears as a white minus-density spot on the film. Normally, this is only a problem with older processors or with processors that need repair. The QCI and QCI-R/T processors were a problem because the rollers were susceptible to damage from Scotch-Brite® pads. Although all processors will give some level of emulsion pick-off, there should be fewer than five spots on an 1824 film.

Recommended Solutions (cont.)

A1—Buff Mark

Objective: To eliminate the buff mark caused by the latest design change to the Kodak developer rack. The buff mark is 1 5/8 in from the leading edge of the film. The kit (see table below) will also help to reduce the pi line artifact that appears 3 1/8 in from the leading edge of the film.

Cause of Problem: The new end plates (Part Nos. 477000 and 477001) with the new guide shoe mounting brackets (Part No. 474596) have increased the distance between the "B" roller and the bottom guide. This directs the leading edge of the film into the second "A" roller, causing the film to hesitate and be buffed by the first "A" roller. The new end plates and brackets do not have enough adjustment to move the film guide within 0.20 in to 0.30 in from the "B" roller. This situation, combined with the reduced traction of the smooth phenolic "B" roller, causes the mark to be created.

Kit contents

This kit is for Kodak processors that have developer racks with the new turnaround end plates (Part Nos. 477000 & 477001) and the new guide shoe mounting brackets (Part No. 474596).

Qty.	Description	Part No.
1	Kodak rubber roller	536884
2	Kodak guide shoe mounting bracket	474596

Note:
The brackets (Part No. 474596) are modified by machining from 0.050 to 0.056 in from the mounting surface. When finished, there will be two different brackets, a right- and a left-hand side. When installed, the film guide will be positioned closer to the "B" roller.

Procedure

1. Remove the developer rack from the processor and rinse with water.
2. Check the large "B" roller; if it is rubber, proceed to step 4.
3. Replace the "B" roller with a rubber "B" roller. The bearings must be removed from the phenolic "B" roller and put into the rubber "B" roller.
4. Remove the bottommost film guide from the rack.
5. Remove the two guide shoe mounting brackets.
6. Install the modified chain-side and gear-side brackets. These brackets will position the film guide closer to the large "B" roller in the turnaround. The trailing edge of the guide should be from 0.020 to 0.030 in from the "B" roller.
7. Install the film guide.
8. Put the rack into the processor and check operation by processing a film.

A2—Buff Mark—DDP—Du Pont Daylight Processor

Objective: To reduce the buff mark to an acceptable level.

Cause of Problem: This common problem usually starts after the developer racks have been removed for cleaning. PROCEDURE: The only solution is to reposition the film guides in the developer rack by bending them into place. This procedure should be performed by a Du Pont service representative.

B1—Pi Line—DDP—Du Pont

Daylight Processor

Objective: To reduce the line(s) on the film.

Artifact Characteristics: One or more lines on the film that are spaced at 3 1/8-in intervals from the leading edge. The lines will not extend from edge to edge. They are more noticeable in reflected light than on a view box.

Procedure: The only solution is to reposition the film guides in the wash and/or developer rack by bending them into place. This procedure should be performed by a Du Pont service representative.

C1—Multiple Bands

A—Kodak Processor

Objective: To reduce or eliminate the problem caused by a swollen bearing in a new or rebuilt developer rack.

Cause of Problem: A swollen bearing in the "D" roller (located just above the large "B" roller) of new or rebuilt developer racks causes the rollers to hesitate, resulting in plus-density marks on the film.

Parts Needed

Qty	Description
1	Sharp, 1/4-in drill bit

Procedure

1. Remove the developer rack and rinse with fresh water.
2. Check the rollers and verify that they are turning without skipping. Watch the three rollers located above the "B" roller (two "E" rollers and a "D" roller).

Note: In extreme cases, the sprocket on the "E" roller will be worn. In some cases, it will break and spin freely on the roller, causing film jams.

3. Remove the "D" roller.
4. Enlarge the two bearings in the "D" roller with a 1/4-in drill bit. (This can normally be done by hand.) The gear end will usually be tighter than the chain idler end.
5. Put the rack together and adjust the drive chain. Do not make the chain too tight or too loose, since either situation will increase the marks.
6. Run a film exposed to a density between 1.0 and 1.8 to check for the appearance of multiple bands.

Notes:
- All racks have some level of plus-density chatter; however, it is normally not as noticeable on a radiograph.
- If the marks are still noticeable, it may be necessary to replace the roller studs. All of the studs on both sides of the developer rack must be replaced. The new studs (Part No. 474477), which are sold in quantities of 36 for approximately $1.00 each, are more susceptible to swelling than the nut-and-screw type (Part No. 470507).

B—QC1 R/T

Objective: To eliminate the plus-density chatter lines across a single-emulsion film.

Cause of Problem: A design deficiency with the R/T.

Procedure

• Order a new developer rack (Part No. 635400-501).

D1—Black Spots

Objective: To eliminate black spots on the film.
Cause of Problem: Worn developer rack produces wet pressure marks that appear as black spots on the film.

Procedure

1. Confirm that the processor is the cause of the problem by processing two films with two different emulsion numbers. The films do not need to be exposed. The marks, which will be quite apparent on films, will be greater along the two edges of the film. If the marks appear on both emulsions, continue with step 2. If not, proceed to step 3.
2. Rebuild or replace the developer rack. (The rebuilt rack must include new bearings, shafts, and end plates, depending on the degree of wear.)
Recommendation: It is quicker and, in most cases, less expensive to simply buy a new rack.
3. If the artifact appears only on one emulsion, discontinue use of the problem emulsion and contact the film representative.

E1—Mottle/Lines—Random

Objective: To eliminate plus-density patterns on exposed film.
Cause of Problem: Dirty, worn, damaged, or defective rollers.
Note: Verify that the developer rack is clean before proceeding.

Procedure

1. Visually inspect the developer rollers to verify that they are not covered with emulsion. The emulsion, which can be seen and felt on the rollers, is most evident on the black rollers.
Note: If films are fed into the processor emulsion up, the center rollers must also be checked.

2. Expose films from two different emulsions to a density between 1.0 and 1.8.
3. Process the films, feeding them into the processor the same way the technicians do.
4. View the films. When the rollers are dirty or covered with emulsion, the left edge of the film will have a definite darker plus-density band approximately 3/8 to 1/2 in wide. If this is the case, proceed to step 5.
5. Clean the rack with a nonabrasive cleaning pad, such as a Scotch-Brite® pad, and thoroughly rinse.

E2—Mottle/Lines—Random or Repetitive

Objective: To reduce plus-density patterns and line artifacts on exposed film to an acceptable level.
Cause of Problem: All plastic rollers in Kodak processors that are not part no. 489693 (for M6B) may cause a pattern on the film. Also, any rollers cleaned with Scotch-Brite® pads may cause line artifacts. These problems result from the developer rack rollers.
Note: Verify that the developer rack is clean before proceeding.

Procedure

1. Expose films from two different emulsions to a density between 1.0 and 1.8.
2. Process the films, feeding them into the processor the same way the technicians do.
3. View the films. If marks appear as mottle or diagonal lines, proceed with steps 4 through 6 below.
4. Remove the developer rack from the processor and rinse with fresh water.
5. Inspect the hard plastic roller surface for imperfections or marks. If you can see or feel patterns on the roller surface, the same pattern is probably on the film. Rollers affected are the "H", "C", and "E" assemblies.
6. Check with the service group that maintains the processor to determine if the rollers are part no. 489693 (for M6B). If they are not, replace all of the "H", "C", and "E" rollers. These rollers are sold separately and in kits (refer to tables below).

Kit No.	Processor
489-798	M6
489-869	M8

Roller No.	Processor	Qty.
489693 (M6B)	M6, M8	16
489693 (M6B)	M7	7

E3—Mottle/Lines—Repetitive

Objective: To reduce repetitive, plus-density patterns on exposed film to an acceptable level.

Cause of Problem: The developer on the surface of the rollers is normally oxidized; if there are pits or depressions in the surface, they will hold concentrations of developer that will image on the film. The image will be repeated more than once and will look just like the nonuniform surface of the roller. Some extremely critical customers complain about the pattern of the rubber rollers, which is mottled and very uniform.

Procedure

1. Inspect the developer to fix crossover rollers. The rollers should be smooth without any imperfections. If the rubber is pitted or damaged, proceed to step 2.
2. Replace the crossover rollers with new rubber rollers. In most cases, new rubber rollers will eliminate the problem.
3. Verify that the problem has been solved by processing films.

Note: In extreme cases, the rollers may have to be replaced with silicon rubber rollers. These rollers are blue-green in color and softer than the black rubber rollers. They are also more expensive than the rubber rollers, costing $250 each.

E4—Mottle/Lines—Konica QX400

Objective: To eliminate the plus-density lines.

Cause of Problem: Some of the processors were assembled with grooved rollers in the developer rack. These rollers produce plus-density patterns on single-emulsion films.

Procedure

1. Inspect the developer rack. All of the rollers should have a smooth surface. Replace all rough or grooved rollers with smooth ones.
2. Check the operation of the rack by processing a film.

F1—Curtain Runback

Objective: To reduce the problem of developer flowing back on the edge of the film. (It cannot be eliminated.)

Cause of Problem: The developer-to-fix crossover nip is not creating a good, tight squeegee action. As a result, the developer flows back on the edge of the film.

Parts Needed

Qty.	Description	Part No.
1	Kodak developer to fix crossover assembly	240057
2	Heavy-duty springs	653776-001

Procedure

1. Expose films to a density between 1.0 and 1.8.
2. Process the films. The artifact will be apparent on the trailing edge of the exposed film.
3. Remove the springs from the new developer to fix crossover assembly and replace with heavy-duty springs (Part No. 653776-001).
4. Remove the developer to fix crossover from the processor.
5. Install the new developer to fix crossover.

F2—Curtain Runback

Parts Needed

Qty.	Description	Part No.
2	Heavy-duty springs	653776-001

Procedure

1. Remove the developer to fix crossover assembly.
2. Verify that the rollers are silicon rubber; then proceed to step 3. If they are not silicon rubber, proceed to F1.
3. Remove the springs and replace them with the heavy-duty springs (Part No. 653776-001).

G1—Water Spots

Objective: To reduce or eliminate the plus- and minus-density spots across the film. (This is only a temporary solution until the vendor can solve this processor problem.)

Cause of Problem: The exit squeegee of the wash rack is leaving water droplets on the film. The manufacturer, AFP, is working to find a solution.

Items Needed

Qty.	Description
2	Jet Dry packets or a similar solution used in dishwashers to eliminate water spotting. (These items are available at most grocery stores.)

Procedure

- Add the packets to the wash tank and replace as needed.

G2—Water Spots

Objective: To eliminate the water-spot pattern on the surface of the films. The pattern can be severe enough to cause plus-density artifacts in the image area.

Cause of Problem: When the center of the 0.75-in rubber roller at the exit nip of the wash rack does not make proper contact with the 1-in roller above it, excessive water is carried through to the dryer rack, resulting in water spots on the film surface.

Solution: Refer to Du Pont Service Bulletin C416-1 (5/11/89).

Procedure

1. Remove the wash rack from the processor.
2. Remove the center 0.75-in rubber roller and retain the roller pins.
3. Locate the center point on the bottom 0.75-in rubber roller. Mark a distance of 1 in from either side of the center point.
4. Using a knife, remove all but the center 2 in of rubber on the roller. It should easily peel off the roller core.
5. Replace the center 0.75-in rubber roller with a new 0.75-in polyurethane roller (Du Pont Part No. 276985-011).

Note: It may be necessary to trim the shoulders on the bearings of the bottom two rollers to guarantee good nip pressure.

H1—White Blotches

Objective: To eliminate minus-density areas from the film.

Cause of Problem: The silver was not exposed to developer because emulsion in the developer was pressed onto the film surface by rollers, thus blocking development. The emulsion is removed in the fix and/or wash, leaving a minus-density spot in the image area. The amount of emulsion in the developer and the severity of the artifact are related to the emulsion run. The increase in emulsion is coming from the edge of the film. In most cases, the problem is caused by fractured emulsion edges on the film. Some emulsions can be worse than others; therefore, changing the emulsion will normally eliminate the problem.

Artifact Characteristics: When viewed with an 8X to 10X magnifier, the artifact will appear as blotchy, minus-density areas across the film. These areas are nonuniform in size and appear in clusters. The center of the white spots at 20X magnification usually have a nonuniform density. Sometimes, there are also black rings that appear in the lower-density areas. These rings may appear to be fingerprints; however, upon closer observation they are seen as black, nonuniform rings.

Procedure

Note: Because the problem is related to the emulsion, it will be necessary to try different emulsion numbers of film. Also, since the problem has not been severe, simply changing to another emulsion number usually eliminates the problem.

1. Check the emulsion number of the film being processed.
2. Thoroughly clean the developer rack.
3. Dump the developer in the processor and replace it with fresh chemistry.
4. Change to another emulsion number. If the problem still occurs, repeat this procedure until the blotches are gone.

I1—Pick-Off

Objective: To eliminate bright white spots across the exposed area of film.

Note: IT IS IMPORTANT TO VERIFY THAT THE PROBLEM IS CAUSED BY THE PROCESSOR AND NOT BY DUST OR DIRT CAUGHT BETWEEN THE FILM AND SCREEN OR A DEFECTIVE SCREEN.

Cause of Problem: Usually a roller is not turning under load because of a defect in the processor racks, such as loose chains or springs. Pick-off can occur in the developer, fix, wash, or dryer racks.

Important: The amount of pick-off can vary depending on the orientation of the emulsion when processed (emulsion up versus emulsion down).

Artifact Characteristics: Appears on the view box as bright white spots across the exposed area of the film. Emulsion pick-off is the removal of emulsion. Under 30X or greater magnification, the area in the white spot will be void of any silver.

Processor Check: White light from two to four films and then process them. Make sure that the films are processed with the emulsion oriented the same way as the technologist orients it because some processors will have more emulsion pick-off when the films are fed emulsion up versus emulsion down. The films will show the level of pick-off that the processor is giving. If the amount of pick-off is greater than five spots per 1824 film, follow the appropriate procedure below.

Procedure

For Kodak and Competitive Processors

1. Verify that the developer rack chain is tight and that all rollers are turning. Severe pick-off only occurs when rollers are hesitating and not turning correctly.
2. Verify that the "D" roller in the developer rack moves freely.
3. Check the fix and wash racks for the same conditions.

For Du Pont Processors: DDP—Du Pont Daylight Processor

1. Verify that all of the springs are in place (especially the turnaround in the developer rack) and that all rollers are turning.
2. Make sure that only DCS-style racks are used and that the earlier-generation racks are not in the processor.

I2—Pick-Off

Objective: To eliminate bright white spots across the exposed area of the film.

Note: IT IS IMPORTANT TO VERIFY THAT THE PROBLEM IS CAUSED BY THE PROCESSOR AND NOT BY DUST OR DIRT CAUGHT BETWEEN THE FILM AND SCREEN OR A DEFECTIVE SCREEN.

Cause of Problem: In many cases, all of the Tinby rollers in the racks have been damaged by an abrasive-type cleaning pad, such as a Scotch-Brite® pad.

Artifact Characterisitics: Appears on the view box as bright white spots across the exposed area of the film. Emulsion pick-off is the removal of emulsion. Under 30X or greater magnification, the area in the white spot will be void of any silver.

Processor Check: White light two to four films and then process them. Make sure that the films are processed with the emulsion oriented the same way as the technologist orients it because some processors will have more emulsion pick-off when the films are fed emulsion up versus emulsion down. The films will show the level of pick-off that the processor is giving. If the amount of pick-off is greater than five spots per 1824 film, follow the appropriate procedure below.

For QC1-R/T or QCI Processors

Parts Needed

Description	Part No.	Stock No.
Top delivery racks	999028002	030147
Rear delivery racks	999028010	

- Replace the racks with the newer DCS style, which is designed to reduce pick-off.

Notes

- All of the racks must be replaced to reduce the level of pick-off to less than five per 1824 film.
- The QC1 dryer cannot be changed to the DCS style and may not yield an acceptable film after changing only the wet racks; therefore, it may be necessary to replace the QC1.

3. Guide to Common Processing Problems— Non–Du Pont Chemistries

MAJOR CAUSES	Base Fog	Contrast		Film Speed		Film Condition			
	Increased	Reduced	Increased	Reduced	Increased	Wet/Damp	Improper Clearing	Dirty	Scratched
DEVELOPER									
Temperature	1	1	1	1	1	3	2	2	2
Depleted	5	1		2		2	2	2	2
Contaminated	4	2		3	1	2	2	2	3
No Starter	2	1			1		5		
Overdiluted		3		3		2	2	2	2
Incorrectly Mixed		1	1	2	2	2	3	2	3
FIXER									
Depleted	4	2			2	1	1	3	2
WASH									
Water Problems								1	
Dirty Water								2	
MECHANICAL									
Dryer Problems						3		3	2
Loss of Circulation		4		5	5	2	2	2	
Dirty Rollers	3	3			3	4		2	4
Misaligned Guideshoes									1
OTHER									
Improper Film Handling					4			3	2
Safelights	2	2			4				
Storage°	2	2			3				
Replenishment Rates Incorrect	4	2	1	2	3	2			
Filter Too Small								2	

1 CHECK FIRST   2 CHECK SECOND   3 CHECK THIRD   4 CHECK FOURTH   5 CHECK LAST

°Film should be stored at 70°F (20°C) and at 40 to 70% relative humidity; film should be rotated first-in first-out method.

4. How to Alter Exposure Factors

Equipment

1. Grid vs. Nongrid
   Grid requires approximately 2.5 times more exposure than nongrid. Increase or decrease accordingly.
2. Stationary grid
   Increased contrast. Requires increased exposure compared with most reciprocating Buckys. Check grid ratio.
3. Collimation
   When coning down, may need to increase exposure from 25 to 35%, due to reducing scatter radiation.
4. Magnification views
   Magnification requires increase in exposure time compared with routine views. Try to keep exposures as low as possible because of reciprocity failure. Try using faster screen. Small focal spot required.
5. Automatic exposure device
   a. May not always compensate for pathologic abnormalities. Go to manual exposure when necessary or try a faster screen.
   b. Equipment is able to compensate for patient thickness; automatically or with density knob control.

Patient

1. Decrease exposure when working with
   a. Adipose patient compressing less than 4.5 cm.
   b. Pendulous breast that flattens to a minimal thickness of breast tissue.
   c. Postmenopausal patient.
   d. Patient who has had multiple pregnancies.
2. Increase exposure when working with
   a. Young, dense breast.
   b. Premenopausal patient with no children.
   c. Lactating breast.
   d. Post-radiation-therapy patients.
   e. Compression greater than 4.5 cm.
   f. Patient who cannot be compressed.
   g. Patient on hormone treatments.

3. Increase kVp when (*Note:* in mammography, the range to increase kVp is very small)
   a. Need to reduce exposure time (to eliminate patient motion).
   b. Necessary to penetrate dense breast.
4. Decrease kVp when
   a. Increasing contrast on the adipose breast.
5. Adipose breast
   a. Decrease kVp to increase contrast.
   b. Reduce mAs if patient compresses less than 4.5 cm.
   c. Increase mAs if patient compresses greater than 4.5 cm.
6. Average patient
   Compensate thickness with mAs.
7. Dense patient
   Will depend on patient's breast tissue composition and thickness. Try to keep kVp as low as possible. Adjust mAs when possible. Go to a faster screen. Alter the target and filtration material.
8. Young dense breast, rock hard
   a. Use a faster screen.
   b. Increase mAs.
   c. Use manual technique.
   d. Cone down to reduce scatter.
   e. Keep kVp as low as possible.
      Molybdenum target: no greater than 30 kVp.
   f. Use an alternate target and filtration (only possible with dual-anode equipment).

Special Cases

1. Implant patients
   Manual technique unless employing the pinch view. With some types of old encapsulated implants, manual exposure preferred.
2. Specimens
   Unless doing whole breast, Bucky not required. Go to nongrid or magnification-nongrid and reduce kVp. Molybdenum target: 22–24 kVp.
3. Anteroposterior views
   Try using higher kVp to reduce patient exposure. Molybdenum target: 34–46 kVp.

Note: The guide above contains suggestions to adjust exposure factors. Consult the user's guide from the mammography equipment manufacturer to determine the best method to alter exposure factors on the control panel.

5. Positioning Problems

Problem	Solution

Problem

1. Deep lesion located laterally. Seen on lateral or mediolateral oblique (MLO) view but not on craniocaudal.

2. Deep lesion located medially.

3. Deep lesion, upper outer quadrant. Seen on contact lateral but not on craniocaudal.

4. Deep lesion, lower inner quadrant.

5. Lesion located deep and high along chest wall. Seen on mediolateral or mediolateral oblique.

6. Lesion deep along chest wall. Difficulty positioning or pulling away.

7. Lesion requiring further evaluation such as reducing patient motion, improving clarity, increasing contrast, spreading of breast tissue.

8. Areas in question, e.g., microcalcifications. Improved detail. Alter patient management.

9. Altering look of suspicious area.

10. Improving detail of lesion located in medial aspect of breast.

11. Evaluating skin calcifications or parenchymal abnormalities.

12. Trying to perform medial lateral oblique on a thin or kyphotic patient.

13. Scar tissue or surgical site.

14. Difficulty compressing patient in craniocaudal projection. Example: male patient.

Note: For further problem solving, see Chapter 7, Section 7.

Solution

1. Exaggerated craniocaudal projection with lateral orientation.

2. Cleavage view or an exaggerated craniocaudal view for medial aspect.
3. Mediolateral oblique or Axillary Tail projection.

4. Cleavage or valley view.

5. Caudocranial or cleavage view.

6. Anteroposterior view, spot compression, coat hanger view, reverse compression device.

7. Spot compression.

8. Magnification views or spot compression.

9. Manipulate exposure factors.

10. Lateral medial—90° lateral, or lateromedial oblique.

11. Tangential view.

12. a. Lateromedial oblique view.
    b. Oblique for upper breast, contact lateral for lower breast.
13. Marking scar with lightweight wire or beebee.

14. Caudocranial view.

6. Parameters to Be Tested for Good Mammography Quality Assurance

I. Technologists QC Procedures

Test Procedure	Frequency	Criteria
Darkroom cleanliness	Daily	NA
PQC startup	Startup	Determine base fog, mid-density, and density difference. Mid-density: step closest to 1.20 Density difference: step closest to 2.20 − step closest to 0.43.
	Daily	Base fog: ≤0.03 Md: ±0.10, caution when >0.10, stop when >0.15 Dd: ±0.10, caution when >0.10, stop when >0.15
Screen cleaning	Weekly	As recommended
Phantom images	Monthly	Background density >1.20, fluctuation permitted ± 0.20 Density difference: approximately 0.40 ± 0.05 Visible objects: Minimum requirement: 4 fibers, 3 micros, 3 masses
Darkroom fog	Semiannually	Density difference ≥0.05
Screen-film contact	Semiannually	>1 cm in diameter black areas after cleaning unacceptable <1 cm in diameter black dots OK if moved after clean
Compression	Semiannually	25 to 40 lb.
Repeat analysis	Quarterly	2% preferred, 5% acceptable retake and repeat rate
View box	Weekly	NA
Analysis of fixer	Quarterly	$<0.05 \text{ g/m}^2$
Visual checklist	Monthly	NA

II. Medical Physicist Test Procedures

Test Procedure	Frequency	Criteria
Mammography unit	Annually	NA
Radiation field/light source	Annually	Radiation field may exceed chest wall edge ≤2% of SID, remaining 3 sides may not exceed the size of the image receptor.
Focal spot size	Annually	Pinhole: 50% of the nominal focal spot Bar Phantom: 13 lp/mm parallel to anode-cathode 11 lp/mm perpendicular anode-cathode
kVp and reproducibility	Annually	±5% of nominal kVp setting
HVL	Annually	≥0.31 mm of Al at 29 kVp; prefer <0.39. See calculation formula for Mo/Rh and Rh/Rh
AEC reproducibility	Annually	±0.30 optical density average over kVp and thickness (2 to 6 cm). If unachievable, make technique chart.
Screen speed	Annually	Optical density maximum permitted is 0.30 w/0.05 deviation
Dose	Annually	<3 mGy or 0.30 rads
Image quality	Annually	Phantom image
Artifact analysis	Annually	Find source and delete

III. Radiologist Responsibilities

Ongoing	Primary responsibility and implementation of QA/QC program.
Ongoing	Provide adequate time in scheduling for QC testing.
Ongoing	Select one technologist to perform QC testing.
Ongoing	Select a medical physicist to perform the physicist QC testing and to oversee the QC testing performed by the technologist.
Ongoing	Responsible for the quality of films produced.

As defined in the 1994 ACR Mammography Quality Control Manual

Appendix

Suggested Needs for a Mammography Room

The needs of each facility will depend upon the procedures performed as well as whether the facility is a screening facility or a diagnostic facility.

A. Dedicated mammography equipment
   1. Dedicated mammography unit
      Optional: Chair or stretcher
      Holder or accessory rack
   2. Cabinet for storage of supplies
   3. Cassettes
      Recommended: From 4 to 18×24 cm and 24×30 cm per technologist per room and/or per x-ray room
   4. Positioning markers
      Left and right:
      • Craniocaudal
      • Mediolateral oblique
      • 90° lateral(s)—mediolateral and laterome-dial lateral
      • Miscellaneous markers for supplemental views
B. Processing
   1. Darkroom
      • Safelight and filter
      • Film bin or plastic film box
      • Processor
      • Chemistry mixer
      • Silver reclaimer
   2. Daylight processing
      • Chemistry mixer
      • Silver reclaimer
   3. Date stickers or date hole puncher
C. View boxes
   1. In mammography room
   2. Processing area
   3. Radiologist reading area
      All view boxes should be of the same color and intensity, appropriate to the size of the radiographs. Care should be taken not to install the view boxes near any windows or extraneous lighting.
D. Patient amenities
   1. Hair spray
   2. Deodorant
   3. Washcloths
   4. Towels
   5. Patient gowns
      Optional: Paper cape gowns with ties in the front
E. Patient education materials
   1. Brochures, to include BSE instruction, miscellaneous information about mastectomy and/or "Reach-to-Recovery" type programs.
   2. Videotapes
   3. VCR and TV
   4. Postmammography instructions
   5. Educational posters
   6. Bulletin board
F. Supplies
   1. History forms
   2. Clipboards

3. Cotton, wool, lintless pads to clean cassettes
4. Antistatic solution
5. Statomatic brush
6. ID camera for marking film (darkroom or x-ray room)
7. Cleaning solution for mammography unit
8. Tape measure and plastic ruler
9. Felt-tip pens: water-soluble or skin-marking
10. BBs or x-spots
11. Thin wire
12. Various tapes: (paper, nylon, hypoallergenic)
13. Scissors
14. Ammonia capsules
15. Small pillows
16. Hot water bottle
17. Metal coat hanger
18. Plastic lids

G. Supplies for special procedures
1. Contrast material, vital dye
2. Sterile gauze pads
3. Betadine
4. Local anesthetic (lidocaine)
5. Syringes (1 cc, 5 cc)
6. Needles (25 g, 23 g, etc.)
7. Alcohol
8. Alcohol pads (prep)
9. Cannulas (ductography kits)
10. Various breast needles (e.g., sizes and types per the radiologist's preference)
11. Biopsy paddles (and light localizer if available); may wish to order extra paddles and custom-made personalized devices
12. Cassette holder (with or without grid) if nongrid work done routinely
13. Sterile towels

H. Stereotactic procedures
1. Adjunctive equipment that must accompany the dedicated mammography machine
2. Various breast biopsy and cytology needles

I. Quality assurance materials
The minimum requirements are
- Thermometer
- Sensitometer
- Densitometer
- Screen-film contact test tool
- Resolution phantom
- Fixer retention test materials
- Notebooks for quality assurance manual(s)

Other facilities may choose to invest in such items as kVp and mAs meters or star pattern.

Bibliography

Alexander FE, Anderson TLJ, Brown HK, et al. The Edinburgh randomised trial of breast cancer screening: Results after 10 years of follow-up. Br J Cancer 1994;70:542–548.

American College of Radiology Committee on Quality Assurance in Mammography. Mammography Quality Control Manual. Reston, VA: American College of Radiology; 1994.

American National Standard Practice for Storate of Processed Safety Photographic Film, ANAI PH 1.43–1981.

Anderson I, Aspegren K, Janzon L, et al. Mammographic screening and mortality from breast cancer: The Malmö mammographic screening trial. BMJ 1988; 297:943–948.

Barnes GT. Radiographic mottle: A comprehensive theory. Med Phys 1982;9:656–667.

Barnes GT, Chakraborty DP. Radiographic mottle and patient exposure in mammography. Radiology 1982;145:815–821.

Barnes GT, Gelskey DE, LaFrance R. A circuit modification that improves mammographic phototimer performance. Radiology 1988;166:773–776.

Bassett L, Gold R. Mammography, Thermography, and Ultrasound in Breast Cancer Detection. New York: Grune & Stratton; 1982.

Bassett LW, Gold RH. Breast radiography using the oblique projection. Radiology 1983;149:585–587.

Bassett L, Gold R: Breast Cancer Detection: Mammography and Other Methods in Breast Imaging, 2nd ed. New York: Grune & Stratton; 1987.

Bassett LW, Gold RH, Gormley L. Positioning in film-screen mammography. Appl Radiol 1988; July: 34-38.

Bassett LW, Gold RH, Kimme-Smith C, et al. Mammographic film-processor temperature, development time, and chemistry: Effect on dose, contrast, and noise. AJR 1989;152:35–40.

Bassett L, Kimme Smith C, Gold R, et al. New mammography screen/film combinations: Imaging characteristics and radiology dose. AJR 1990;154:713–719.

Bernstein F, Sheid CC, Wilson CR. The effect of target composition, kVp, and filtration on patient skin dose and contrast in mammography. Appl Radiol 1977; Jan–Feb:63–69.

Boice JD, Bond VP, Dodd G, et al. Mammography. Bethesda, MD: National Council of Radiological Publications; NCRP report 66, 1985.

Brodie I, Gutcheck. Radiographic information theory and application to mammography. Med Phys 1982;9:79–95.

Burhenne LJW, Hislop TG, Burhenne HJ. The British Columbia Mammography Screening Program: Evaluation of the first 15 months. AJR 1992;158:45–49.

Burkhart RL. A Basic Quality Assurance Program for Small Diagnostic Radiology Facilities. Rockville, MD: HHS Publication FDA; FDA #83-8218, 1983.

Busby RC, Eklund GW, Job JS, Miller SH. Improved imaging of the augmented breast. AJR 1988;151:469–473.

Case C, ed. The Breast Cancer Digest. 2nd ed. Bethesda, MD: US Department of Health and Human Services; 1984.

Chaglassian TA, Dershaw DD. Mammography after prosthesis placement for augmentation or reconstructive mammoplasty. Radiology 1989;170:69–74.

Chan EC. Psychosocial issues in breast disease. Clin Obstet Gynecol 1982;25:447–454.

Chiles JT, Haus AG, Metz CE, Rossman, K. The effect of x-ray spectra from molybdenum and tungsten target tubes on image quality in mammography. Radiology 1976;118:705–709.

Christensen EE, Curry TS, Dowdey JE. An Introduction to the Physics of Diagnostic Radiology. Philadelphia: Lea & Febiger; 1978:2.

Collette HJA, Day NE, Rombach JJ, deWaard F. Evaluation of screening for breast cancer in a non-randomized study (The DOM Project) by means of case control study. Lancet 1984;1:1224–1226.

Cullinan JE, Haus AG. Screen film processing systems for medical radiography: A historical review. RadioGraphics 1989;9:1203–1224.

Curpen BN, Sickles EA, Sillitto RA, et al. The comparative value of mammographic screening for women 40–49 years old versus women 50–64 years old. AJR 1995;164:1099–1103.

Davis SP, Meyer JE, Stomper PC, Weidner N. Suture calcification mimicking recurrence in the irradated breast: A potential pitfall in mammographic evaluation. Radiology 1989;172:247–249.

Day JL, Lightfoot DA, Stanton L, Villafana T. Dosage evaluation in mammography. Radiology 1984;150:577–584.

Dean PB, Tabar L. Quality aspects in mammography. Medicamundi 1984;29:71–75.

Degenshein GA, Ceccarelli F. The history of breast cancer surgery. Breast 1984;3(2):34,43.

DePeredes ES. Atlas of Film-Screen Mammography. Baltimore, MD: Urban & Schwarzenberg; 1989.

Dershaw D, Materson ME, Malik S, Cruz N. Mammography using an ultra high strip density stationary, focused grid. Radiology 1985;156:541–544.

DeWerd LA. Mammography Quality Assurance. Med Med Electr 1988;19:94–98.

Duffy SW, Kirkpatrick AE, Muir BB, Roberts MM. Oblique-view mammography: Adequacy for screening. Radiology 1984;151:39–41.

Eastgate RJ, Ergun DL, Jennings RJ, Siedband MP. Optimal x-ray spectra for screen-film mammography. Med Phys 1981;8:629–639.

Eddy DM, Hasselblad V, Hendee W, McGivney W. The value of mammography screening in women under the age of 50 years. JAMA 1988;259:1512–1519.

Egan RL. Mammography. Springfield, IL: Charles C Thomas; 1964.

Egan RL. Breast Imaging, 3rd ed. Baltimore, MD: University Park Press; 1984.

Egan RL. Breast cancer screening. Admin Radiol 1987;Oct:14–18.

Egan RL. Breast Imaging: Diagnosis and Morphology of Breast Diseases. Philadelphia: Saunders; 1988.

Egan RL, McSweeney M. Grids in mammography. Radiology 1983;146:359–362.

Ehrlich SM, Feig SA, Haus AG, et al. Mammography screening: Technology, radiation dose and risk, quality control, and benefits to society. Radiology 1990;174:627–656.

Eklund GW. Innovations in mammographic compression. AJR 1988;150:791–792.

Eklund GW, Surratt D. Extended developer processing time. Admin Radiol 1989;April:22–23.

Eklund GW, Carenosa G. The art of mammographic positioning. Radiol Clin North Am 1992; 3:21–53.

Erickson L, Haus AG. Image quality factors and radiation dose in mammography. J Imaging Technol 1984;10:29–35.

Feig S. Decreased breast cancer mortality through mammographic screening: Results of clinical trials. Radiology 1988;167:659–665.

Feig SA. Radiation risk from mammography. Is it clinically significant? AJR 1984;143:469–475.

Feig SA. Xero and screen-film: Mammography's rival systems. Diagn Imaging 1987; Sept:112–118.

Feig SA. The importance of supplementary mammographic views to diagnostic accuracy. AJR 1988;151:40–41.

Feig SA, McLelland R. Breast Carcinoma. New York: Masson; 1983.

Feig SA, Karasick S, Koople HA, et al. Clinical applications of yttrium filters for exposure reduction. RadioGraphics 1984;4:479–505.

Feig SA, Haus AG, Jans RG, et al. Mammography: A User's Guide. Bethesda, MD: National Council on Radiation Protection; NCRP report 85, 1986.

Fox SA, Klos DS, Tsou CV. Underuse of screening mammography by family physicians. Radiology 1988;166:431–433.

Georgiade NG, Georgiade GS, Riefkohl R. Aesthetic Surgery of the Breast. Philadelphia: Saunders; 1990.

Gershon-Cohen J. Historical review. Breast Roentgenol 1961;86:879–883.

Gray JE. Quality Assurance in Diagnostic Radiology, Nuclear Medicine and Radiation Therapy. Rockville, MD: Department of Health, Education and Welfare; 1976.

Gray JE, Frank ED, Stears J, Winkler NT. Quality Control in Diagnostic Imaging: A Quality Control Cookbook. Baltimore: University Park Press; 1983.

Groenenstein M, van der Zwagg H. New films, lower mammogram dose while maintaining image quality. Diagn Imaging 1988; April:131—132.

Hall DA, Johnson LL, Kelley JE, et al. Comparison of two screen-film combinations in contact and magnification mammography: Detectability of microcalcifications. Radiology 1988;168:657–659.

Harper P. Ultrasound Mammography. Baltimore: University Park Press; 1985.

Harrill C, White S, Gillespie K, et al. Evaluation of a dual- screen. AJR 1989;152:483–486.

Harris JR, Hellman S, Henderson IC, Kinne DW. Breast Diseases. Philadelphia: Lippincott; 1987.

Haus AG. Recent Trends in Screen-Film Mammography. Rochester, NY: Eastman Kodak; 1984.

Haus AG. Screen-Film Mammography Update. Rochester, NY: Eastman Kodak; 1984;486.

Haus AG. Trends in Screen-Film Mammography. Rochester, NY: Eastman Kodak; 1986.

Haus AG, Erickson L. Image quality factor and radiology dose in mammography. J Imaging Technol 1984;10:29–35.

Haus AG. Technologic improvements in screen-film mammography. Radiology 1990;174;628–637.

Haus AG. Advances in screen-film mammography improve image quality, lower dose. Product Dev 1987;1–3.

Haus AG, Tabar L. Processing of mammographic films: Technical and clinical considerations. Radiology 1989;173:65–69.

Haus AG, Metz C, Chiles J, Rossman K. The effect of x-ray spectra from molybdenum and tungsten target: Tubes on image quality in mammography. Radiology 1976;118:705–709.

Health Sciences Markets Division. The Fundamentals of Radiology, 12th ed. Rochester, NY: Eastman Kodak; 1980.

Hwkcuwq MA, Heang-Ping C. et al: Breast thickness in routine mammograms—Effect on image quality and radiation dose. AJR 1994; 163: 1371–1374.

Hendrick, RE. Standardization of image quality and radiation dose in mammography. Radiology. 1990;174:648–654.

Hogan B. The image of mammography. Admin Radiol 1990;Feb:32–35.

Holland R. The role of specimen x-ray in the diagnosis of breast cancer. Diagn Imaging 1985;54:178–185.

Holleb AI. Restoring Confidence in Mammography. New York: American Cancer Society; 1976.

Homer MJ. Breast imaging. Pitfalls, controversies, and some practical thoughts. Radiol Clin North Am 1985;23:459–472.

Homer MJ. Myths about mammography: A Patient Education Feature. Prime Care Cancer. 1986;June:53–56.

Homer MJ, Pile-Spellman ER. Needle localization of nonpalpable breast lesions: The importance of communication. Appl Radiol 1987; November:88–98.

Hutchinson GB, Shapiro S. Lead time gained by diagnostic screening for breast cancer. J Natl Cancer Inst 1968;41:665–681.

Ikeda DM, Sickles EA. Second-screening mammography: One versus two views per breast. Radiology 1988;168:65–656.

Jackson VP, Lex AM, Smith DJ. Patient discomfort during screen-film mammography. Radiology 1988;168:421–423.

Jakobsson S, Lundgren B. Single view mammography: A simple and efficient approach to breast cancer screening. Cancer 1976;38:1124–1129.

Jenkins D. Radiographic Photography and Imaging Processes. Baltimore: University Park Press; 1980.

Jennings RJ, Eastgate RJ, Siedband MP, Ergun DL. Optimal x-ray spectra for screen film mammography. Med Phys 1981;8:629–639.

Kimme-Smith C, Wang J, Debruhl N, et al: Mammograms obtained with rhodium vs molybdenum anodes: Contrast and dose differences. AJR 1994;162:1313–1317.

Kirkpatrick AE, Law J. A comparative study of film and screens for mammography. Br J Radiol 1987;60:73–78.

Kopans DB. Breast Imaging. Philadelphia: Lippincott; 1989.

Kopans DB, Meyer JE. Breast physical examination by the mammographer. Appl Radiol 1983; March/April:103–106.

Kopans DB, Meyer JE, Sadowsky N. Breast imaging. N Engl J Med 1984;310:960–967.

Kowalczyk N. Patients' perceptions of a mammographic examination. Radiol Technol 56(4):212–215.

Lamel DA, Brown RF, Shaver JW, et al. The Correlated Lecture Laboratory Series in Diagnostic Radiological Physics. Rockville, MD: HHS Publication FDA; 1981; vol. 8150.

Lawrence DJ. A simple method of processor control. Med Radiol Photogr 1973;49:2–6.

Leborgne R. Diagnosis of tumors of the breast by simple roentgenographe: Calcifications in carcinomas. Am J Roentgenol Radium Ther 1951;65:1–11.

Letton AH, Mason EM, Wilson JP. The value of breast screening in women less than fifty years of age. Cancer 1977;40:1–3.

Linden SS, Sickles EA. Sedimented calcium in benign breast cysts: The full spectrum of mammographic presentations. AJR 1989;152:967–971.

Lippman ME, Lichter AS, Danforth DN. Diagnosis and Management of Breast Cancer. Philadelphia: Saunders; 1988.

Lofgren M, Andersson I, Lindholm K. Stereotactic fine needle aspiration for cytologic diagnosis of nonpalpable breast lesion. AJR 1990;154:1191–1195.

Logan WW. Screen-Film Mammography. New York: Grune & Stratton; 1982:61–72.

Logan WW, Muntz EP. Screen-film mammography technique: Compression and other factors, in: Reduced Dose Mammography. New York: Masson; 1979;418–419.

Martin JE. Atlas of Mammography: Histologic and Mammographic Correlations, 2nd ed. Baltimore: Williams & Wilkins; 1988:55.

McLelland R. Mammography 1984: Challenge to radiology. AJR 1984;143:1–4.

McLelland R, Hendrick RE, Zinninger M, Wilcox P. The American College of Radiology Accreditation Program. Submitted to the American Journal of Roentgenology, March 1991.

McLelland R. Responding to the challenge of breast cancer screening. Diagn Imaging 1986; June:69–81.

McLemore JM: Quality Assurance in Diagnostic Radiology. Chicago: Year Book Medical; 1981.

Mettlin C, Smart CR, Breast cancer detection guidelines for women aged 40–49 years: Rationale for the American Cancer Society Reaffirmation of Recommendations. CA 1994 44:248–255.

Meschan I. Radiographic Positioning and Related Anatomy. Philadelphia: Saunders; 1968.

Michigan Department of Public Health—Division of Radiologic Health. Recommendations for Mammography Facility. Ann Arbor, MI: November 1988: RH-874.

Moskowitz M. Diagnostic categorical course in breast imaging. Presented at 72nd Scientific Assembly and Annual Meeting of the Radiological Society of North America; Cincinnati, OH: December 1986.

Mulvaney JA. Medical Imaging and Instrumentation '84. The Society of Photo-Optical Instrumentation Engineers, 1984;486.

National Cancer Program. Manual of Procedures and Operations for the National Cancer Institute and the American Cancer Society. Bethesda, MD: US DHEW;1977;vol. 2.

Nielsen B. Scattered Radiation in Diagnostic Radiology. Linkoping, Sweden: Department of Radiation Physics; 1985:vol 196.

Nishikawa RM, Yaffe MJ. Signal to noise properties of mammographic film-screen systems. Med Phys 1985;12:32–39.

Nystrom L, Rutqvist LE, Wall S, et al. Breast cancer screening with mammography: Overview of Swedish radomised trials. Lancet 1993;341:947–978.

Peterson N. Reducing the risk of breast cancer. McCall's 1989; Sept:101–102, 107–108.

Peters ME, Scanlon KA, Voegeli DR, eds. Handbook of Breast Imaging. New York: Churchill Livingstone; 1989.

Porrath S. A Multimodality Approach to Breast Imaging. Rockville, MD: Aspen Publishers; 1986.

Rimer B. Why women resist screening mammography: Patient-related barriers. Radiology 1989; July:243–246.

Robinson AE, Schoenberger SG, Sutherland CM. Breast neoplasms: Duplex sonographic imaging as an adjunct in diagnosis. Radiology 1988;168:665–668.

Rueter FG. Next 1985 Project. Frankfort, KY: Office of the Executive Secretary; 1987.

Sadowsky NL, Feig SA, McLelland R. Breast Imaging: A Guide for Clinicians. Reston, VA: American College of Radiology, Categorical Course; October 1990, Nashville, TN.

Schmidt RA, Vyborny CJ. Mammography as a radiographic examination: An overview. Radiographics 1989;9:723–764.

Schutte HE. Mammography Today. New York; Karger; 1985.

Seago K. Screening mammography: The pressures for reimbursement. Appl Radiol 1986; June/July:17–24.

Seidman H, Gelb S, Silverberg E, et al. Survival experience in the breast cancer detection demonstration project. CA 1987; 37:258–290.

Seidman H. Screening for breast cancer in younger women. CA 1977;27:66–87.

Shapiro S. Evidence on screening for breast cancer from a randomized trial. Cancer 1977;39:2772–2782.

Shapiro S, Strax P, Venet L. Evaluation of periodic breast cancer screening with mammography. JAMA 1966;195:731–738.

Shapiro S, Strax P, Venet L. Presymptomatic Detection and Early Diagnosis. London: Pitman; 1968.

Shapiro S, Strax P, Venet L, Venet W. Adequacies and inadequacies of breast examinations by physicians. Cancer 1969;21:1187–1191.

Shimkin MB. Screening by mammography. JAMA 1966;195:775.

Sickles EA. American College of Radiology statement on screening mammography for women 40–49. ACR Bull 4–93.

Sickles EA. Further experience with microfocal spot magnification mammography in the assessment of clustered breast microcalcifications. Radiology 1980;137:9–14.

Sickles, EA. Efforts to lower dose and maximize diagnostic accuracy. Presented at the 20th National Conference on Breast Cancer; New Orleans; March 15, 1982.

Sickles EA. Breast calcifications: Mammographic evaluation. Radiology 1986;160:289–293.

Sickles EA. Dedicated mammography equipment. Presented at ACR Categorical Course on Mammography; Los Angeles; September 1984.

Sickles EA. The Radiologic Clinics of North America. Philadelphia: Saunders; 1987:vol. 25.

Sickles EA. Practical solutions to common mammo-

graphic problems: Tailoring the examination. AJR 1988:151:31–39.

Sickles EA, Weber WN. High-contrast mammography with a moving grid: Assessment of clinical utility. AJR 1986;146:1137–1139.

Stanton L, Villafana T, Day J, Lightfoot DA. Dosage evaluation in mammography. Radiology 1984;150:57–584.

Strax P, Venet L, Shapiro S. Value of mammography in reduction of mortality from breast cancer in mass screening. AJR 173;117:686–689.

Tabar L, Dean PB. Teaching Atlas of Mammography. New York: Thieme-Stratton; 1983.

Tabar L, Fagerberg G, Duffy SW, et al. Update of the Swedish two-country program of mammographic screening for breast cancer. Radiol Clin North Am 1992;30:187–210.

Thunberg SJ: The effect of different anode/filter combinations on image quality and glandular dose. Prepublication manuscript. August 1994.

Townsend CM. Clinical Symposia: Breast Lumps. Summit, NJ: CIBA Pharmaceutical Company; 1980:32.

U.S. Department of Health and Human Services, Public Health Service, Agency for Health Care Policy and Research. Quality Determinants of Mammography. Rockville MD: AHCPR Publication No 95-0632, October 1994.

U.S. Department of Health, Education, and Welfare. Final Reports of National Cancer Institute ad hoc Committee Working on Mammography Screening for Breast Cancer and a Summary of Their Joint Findings and Recommendations. Bethesda, MD: US DHEW; 1977;vol 1.

Verbeek, ALM, Hendriks JHCL, Holland R, et al. Reduction of breast cancer mortality through mass screening with modern mammography: First results of the Nijmegen Project 1975–1981. Lancet 1984;1:1222– 1224.

Walker E. Mammography. Linking the referring physician. Admin Radiol 1987; March:16–18.

Watt, CA. Quality assurance in mammography and the ACR accreditation program. ACR Categorical Course on Breast Imaging. Nashville, TN: Oct. 1990.

Wayrynen RE. Fundamental Aspects of Film-Screen Systems and Film Processing. Wilmington, DE: EI du Pont de Nemours and Company;

Wellings SR, Jensen HM, Marcum RG. An atlas of subgross pathology of the human breast with special reference to possible precancerous lesions. J Natl Cancer Inst 1975;2:231–273.

Witten DM. The Breast. Chicago: Year Book; 1969.

Wolfe JN. Risk for breast cancer development determined by mammographic parenchymal pattern. Cancer 1976;37:2486–2492.

Zamenhof RG, Homer MJ. I. Equipment mammography: Physical principles. Appl Radiol 1984; September/October:86–99.

Zamenhof RG, Homer MJ. II. Evaluation of equipment and guidelines for quality assurance. Appl Radiol 1984; November/December:51.

Index

Index